Six Strands
of the Web

Six Strands
of the Web

An In-depth Study of the Six Stages of Disease
In Traditional Chinese Medicine

Dr. James Michael Moore

authorHOUSE®

AuthorHouse™
1663 Liberty Drive
Bloomington, IN 47403
www.authorhouse.com
Phone: 1-800-839-8640

Published by AuthorHouse   06/08/2012

ISBN: 978-1-4772-0874-8 (sc)
ISBN: 978-1-4772-0873-1 (hc)
ISBN: 978-1-4772-0872-4 (e)

Library of Congress Control Number: 2012909206

Contents

About the Author

Dr. James Michael Moore OMD was born in 1950. He began his studies in Chinese medicine in 1963. His degrees include: a doctor of naturopathic medicine from Pacific College in Palto Alto, California, in 1980, Master of Acupuncture from the Occident Institute of Chinese Studies in Miami, Florida in 1981, and a Doctorate on Oriental Medicine from Southwest Acupuncture College in Santa Fe, New Mexico in 1988. From 1985-1991, He studied under private tutorship (Chinese herbal medicine) with the late Dr. Hong-yen Hsu at the Oriental Healing Arts Institute in Long Beach, California.

Dr. Moore, a well-respected professional, is known throughout the nation for his healing skills and teaching talents. He has been practicing Chinese medicine full time since 1975 and has been a key figure in his professional community promoting the growth of Chinese medicine. He was the founding president of the Acupuncture Association of New Mexico and served as a member of the New Mexico State Board of Acupuncture for seven years. Dr. Moore was the co-founder, teacher, and assistant director for the Institute of Traditional Medicine and the Southwest Acupuncture College. From 2001-2005 Dr. Moore taught at the Green Mountain Institute of Oriental Medicine, in White Fish, Vermont and was the Department Head for the herbal program. In 2006 he retired from teaching. Presently, Dr. Moore has his practice in Ronan, Montana since 2005.

About This Book

The title of this book reminds us that the study of Chinese medicine is a vast amount of knowledge acquired over thousands of years. The "six stages of disease model" presented here is just six little strands of knowledge in a huge web of understanding of how our bodies deal with disease. This book gives us a close look at how the ancient Chinese viewed the progression of disease. The six stages of disease are like a micro life cycle and battle in which our bodies are fighting the disease process.

This book is designed for the serious student of Chinese medicine. Both the beginner and advanced practitioner will find this information useful from school to everyday clinical practice. The first section of the book covers a basic history and evolution of the six stages of disease. Chapter Two reviews various theoretical concepts related to the six stages. Symptoms and treatment concepts, according to the Chinese classic Shang Han Lun, are examined in Chapter Three.

In Chapter Four complications of combined and overlapping stages of disease show how disease many times will not follow the normal progression of the Six Stage Model. An in- depth study of conformations and the basic treatment concepts for each of the stages are presented in Chapter Five. A quick overview of the twenty-four basic classifications of Chinese herbal formulas will be found in Chapter Six. Primary herbs for each stage and their related formulas are examined in Chapter Seven. Chapter Eight deals with differential diagnosis of syndromes and treatment. Conformations for formulas and a comparison to other formulas from the Classic *Shang Han Lun* (Treaties on Fever and Chills) and the *Jen Kuei Yao Lue*

(Perceptions from the Golden Chamber) are the main emphasis in Chapter Nine.

Practitioners will find Chapter Ten a very useful clinical reference of all ninety herbal formulas (in table form) found in this book. In Chapter Eleven, there are four major lists dealing with the names of individual herbs. The first three lists are a cross reference for herbs listed by the Pin Yin, Pharmaceutical, and Common names. The fourth list gives the classification and function of the 118 herbs used in this work.

Notice

The following information in this book on Chinese herbal formulas is widely used around the world. This information compiled from traditional medical texts and the observations of authorities on Chinese medicine is presented here for its educational value and should not be used to diagnosis, treatment, or prevention of disease without the advice of a properly trained physician or healthcare practitioner.

Preface

The "six stages of disease" and the ancient herbal formulas found in the Classics *Shang Han Lun* (Treatise on Chills and Fever) and *Jen Kuei Yao Lue* (Prescriptions from the Golden Chamber) are still important study material for "Modern Times". These herbal prescriptions have proven themselves as being safe and effective for a wide range of disorders.

Doctor *Zhang Zhongjing's* model for "Six Stages of Disease" is useful not only for fever related disorders, it can be used to help differentiate which formulas may be employed for a great number of health complaints.

It is important to note that the English name for the formulas are from Dr. *Hong-yen Hsu's* works, as he was my mentor for many years. Doctor *Hsu's* English version for each formula is usually made up of the names of its principle herbs, which can be useful in understanding the energetics of the combination or formula in general. Second the Chinese name is given in pin-yin followed by the older style of Wade-Giles in parentheses. The underlined English name version is the literal translation most commonly used today.

Chapter One
History of Six Stages of Disease Model

Overview

The main emphasis in this section is on the history and development of Chinese medicine and its spread to other countries.

- History and evolution of "six stages of disease model"
- *Huangdi's* Internal Classic, or *Huangdi's* Cannon of Medicine
- *Shang Han Lun* (Treatise on Chills and Fever)
- *Jen Kuei Yao Lue* (Prescriptions from the Golden Chamber)
- Japanese *Kanpo*

The Six Stages of Disease *(Liu Jing Bian Zheng)*

Introduction

The "Six Stages of Disease" is a theoretical concept that can be used as a model to help understand the progression and treatment of disease. The pathology of febrile related disorders according to the *Shang Han Lun* (Treatise on Chills and Fever) and *Jen Kuei Yao Lue* (Prescriptions from the Golden Chamber) show how a disease can move from what is known as the surface" or "external" aspect of the body to the "interior" aspect in six major levels each having its own unique pathology and Treatment Concept. The order of these levels of penetration or stages of disease is classified as *taiyang* (greater yang), *shaoyang* (lesser yang), *yangming* (sunlight yang), *taiyin* (greater yin), *shaoyin* (lesser yin), and jueyin (absolute yin). The *jueyin* stage of disease, as it nears its end, is that stage where the body no longer has enough strength to control the balance of *yin* and *yang*. When the body becomes too weak to maintain proper balance of *yin* and *yang*, the disease has won the struggle.

The original Chinese model used to describe the progression of fever related disease was first recorded in the medical classic *Huangdi Nei Jing* (*Huangdi's Internal Classic*, or *Huangdi's Cannon of Medicine*). This is the oldest and greatest Chinese medical classic known. Its authorship is ascribed to the Yellow Emperor *Huangdi* (2698-2589 B.C.). The work was actually written by unknown authors during the Warring States Period (475-221 B.C.).

Huangdi Nei Jing has two parts: *Su Wen* (Plain Questions) and *Ling Shu* (Spiritual Pivot or Divine Axis). In the *Su Wen* chapter 31 ["The Fever", the evolution of disease and how it relates to the "Energetic Layers" of the body is discussed], which states:

> *"The fever generally happens unexpectedly after a shock from Cold. The Taiyang (Small Intestine and Bladder) meridian is attacked first. This meridian of the Taiyang is in connection with the point Fungfu, (Du-16), meeting point of the meridians of the Bladder, the Yang Wei (extra meridian), and the Governor Vessel. This last is so named because it governs the Yang of all the body. The energy of the Tai Yang meridian*

begins at the point Jingming (Bl-1). It is the point therefore which commands all of the Yang energy. If the shock from Cold attacks solely the Yang, even if the temperature is very high, the sick person will not be in danger, but if it simultaneously attacks the Yang and the Yin, the sick person will inevitably be in danger of death.

If the shock from Cold attacks only the Yang:
The first day it is the meridians of the Taiyang (Small Intestine and Bladder) which are attacked, the sick person presents pains at the head and neck; the lumbar region and the vertebral column are stiff, aching all over.

The second day, it is the meridians of the Yangming which are attacked (Large Intestine and Stomach); these meridians passing near the nose and eyes, the sick person presents fever, with a feeling of pain at the eyes, and of dryness of the nose; he cannot sleep peacefully, he is agitated.

The third day, it is the Shaoyang (Triple Burner and Gall Bladder). These meridians passing on the side of the body and to the ears, the chest, and in addition he does not hear well. At this period of the sickness, all the Yang meridians are attacked, but not yet the internal organs. If one makes the sick person perspire, he will be cured, otherwise:

On the fourth day, the illness attacks the Yin meridians beginning with Taiyin (Lung and Spleen). These meridians passing on the abdomen and toward the upper part of the chest, the sick person presents abdominal swelling and dryness of the upper respiratory tracts.

On the fifth day, the illness passes to the Shaoyin meridians (Heart and Kidneys). These meridians passing on the chest and toward the tongue (the Kidney meridian, through a secondary vessel, reaches the point Lien-Chuan (CV-23), the sick person presents dryness of the mouth and tongue: he will be very thirsty.

On the sixth day, the illness passes to the Jueyin meridians (Pericardium and Liver). These meridians passing near the genital parts and reaching the Liver, the sick person presents malaise, and his scrotum is retracted. At this moment of the evolution of the sickness, the Three Yang meridians, the Three Yin meridians, the Six Bowels and the Five Organs have been attacked; the energy and the blood no longer function, this is death.

If, as we have just seen, the Yang meridians and the Yin meridians have not been attacked at the same time, but one after another, and if one has undertaken the correct treatment, one sees the following symptoms appear:

The seventh day, the Taiyang meridians are appeased, and the sick person have less pain at the head and neck.

The eighth day, the Yangming meridians are appeased, and the fever come down.

The ninth day, the Shaoyang meridians are appeased, and the sick person hearing improves.

The tenth day, the Taiyin meridians are appeased, and the sick person recover his appetite.

The eleventh day, the Shaoyin meridians are appeased, and the sick person have less thirst.

The twelfth day, the Jueyin meridians are appeased, and the scrotum is relaxed and soon the cure will be complete.

In order to bring about this cure, it is necessary to provoke perspiration during the first
Three days, and then it is necessary to purge on the fourth.

The Emperor Huangdi (question):
If the Yang and the Yin meridians are affected at the same time, what will the symptoms be?

Chi Po (answer):
If the Taiyang and the Shaoyin meridians are attacked at the same time, the sick person, The first day, pains at the head, dryness of the mouth, and fullness in all the body.

If Yangming and the Taiyin meridians are attacked at the same time, he presents the second day, fullness of the abdomen, loss of appetite, delirium.

If the Shaoyang and the Jueyin meridians are attacked at the same time, he presents the third day, auditory disturbances, and retraction of the scrotum. He can no longer swallow anything: He is in a coma. His death will arrive unexpectedly the six day.

The Emperor Huangdi:
Why does he still survive for three days?

The Physician answers:
The Yangming meridian is the meridian which has the most blood and energy; it
is thanks to it that, even in the coma, the sick person's life can yet be prolonged for
three days."[1]

Over eighteen hundred years ago, (two hundred years after the *Huangdi Nei Jing*), a Chinese medical practitioner, *Zhang Zhongjing*, used the "Six Stages" concept of pathology to explain what he saw as an entire life cycle compressed into a very short span of time. Within this cycle various conformations (syndromes) relating to each stage could be made so that the correct herbal prescription could be used. The conformations for each of the various stages depend not only on the etiology of the disease but also the overall constitution of the individual and how the body is dealing with the disease at the time. After studying and synthesizing the medical writings of his time, *Zhang Zhongjing* developed his concepts of the Six Stages of Disease. This was an elaborate, logical, and practical model, from which, febrile disease caused by "pernicious influences" entering the body could be mapped out and treated. With this model, disease usually follows an orderly progression from the first stage to the last; however, a disease can go straight to any stage, skip stages, or even move in the reverse.

---

[1]   Occidental Institute of Chinese Studies Alumni Association, "The *Nei Ching* (Chinese Medical Classics)", Pg. 81-83 Miami, Florida, (1979)

Chart 1 (Progression of the six stages)

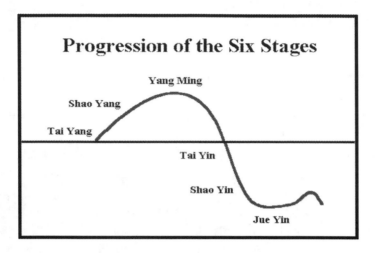

The result of *Zhang Zhongjing's* studies and observations were recorded in his two books *Shang Han Lun* (Treatise on Chills and Fever) and *Jen KueiYao Lue* (Prescriptions from the Golden Chamber). Originally these two were bound together as a single book, but during the *Sung* dynasty (960-1279) they were separated. Historically, when authors cited passages from the *Shang Han Lun*, they were referring to both books. For the purpose of this work *"Shang Han Lun"* will be used to refer to both books. The concepts and approach to dealing with disease found in these two classics are unique.

There is nothing in Western medicine quite like them and yet this form of combating febrile disorders has been used for hundreds of years in the Orient with great success and without the dangerous side effects so common with Western allopathic medicine. With the growing concern about today's super strong medications there is a need for safe alternative medical care that has been proven effective. Traditional Chinese herbal formulas discussed here have been used for centuries without major side effects when properly used.

Development of Chinese Medicine

Prior to Shang Han Lun

Long before recorded Chinese history, the works of the great Emperor *Yen (Shen Nung)* were preserved and handed down verbally from one generation to the next. It is said that *Shen Nung*, who was born over 5,400 years ago, taught the people how to raise crops, rear domestic animals, and test and identify various herbs. Archeological evidence has revealed that *Shen Nung* lived in the regions along the Yellow *(Yangzi)* and *Xiang* river basins. He is known as the "God of Husbandry" and his work was recorded in various historical references such as the following:

Si-Ma Jien's The Historical Records: *"Shen Nung tasted various herbs and determined their medical property and value."*

Hui Nan Zi records: *"When Shen Nung taught the people to taste various herbs, seventy species of poisonous ones were encountered in a single day; hence medical science progressed rapidly."*[2]

Although *Shen Nung's* birth and death cannot be accurately verified, legend has it that while living in *Yuwang* he served eight Lords for 820 years. From this it is believed that 3494 B.C. was the time period of the first truly great pharmacologist of the world.

Approximately 830 years later, another great in Chinese medical history, The Yellow Emperor *(Huangdi)*, became known to the Chinese world. The Yellow Emperor's name was *Gong-Sun Xien Yua.* He is known by the Chinese as the ancestor of the Chinese race. There are a great number of inventions and discoveries attributed to *Huangdi* and he is known as the legendary founder of Chinese medical science.

---

[2] Chen's History of Chinese Medical Science by H. Hsu and W. Peacher pg 3

Research has shown that in the time of *Huangdi* there were only hieroglyphics invented by *Sang Ji*. This form and style of writing of the *Nei Jing* could not have been from the same time period. Many historians throughout the centuries relate the wording and sentence structure of the *Nei Jing* to the time period between that of the Warring States to the beginning of the *Han* Dynasty (403-206 B.C.). This means that there is a time period of 1,271 years between the writing of the *Nei Jing* and the Yellow Emperor. This however, does not reduce the importance of this classic on internal medicine whose contents include ancient physiology, pathology, therapeutics, classification of diseases, systems of meridians, as well as Chinese philosophy.

The four basic diagnostic methods of "observation, listening, questioning, and palpation" in Chinese medicine were originated by *Bian Que* (about 407-310 B.C.). *Bian Que*, originally named *Qin Yueren*, was the first noted medical expert in the period of the Warring States (403-221B.C.) to be recorded practicing acupuncture. Historical Records tell about one of his famous cases:

While out walking one day with his disciples *Tzu Yang* and *Tzu Pao*, *Bian Que* noticed that many people were outside the Emperor's gate offering sacrifices for the Emperor's son who had suddenly become unconscious. After inquiring about the cause and symptoms of the Emperor's son's disease, *Bian Que* sent word to the Emperor "There is still some hope for your son, and I would like to treat him." Examination of the son revealed weak breath and some warmth still inside the legs. *Bian Que* then administered several needles to the head, chest, and limbs whereupon the patient regained his consciousness. With the aid of herbal soups and warming therapy the Emperor's son gradually sat up in bed and regained his health in about 20 days.

Bian Que is reported to have traveled far and wide treating people and alleviating suffering all his life. He was greatly loved and adored for his willingness to help the sick and was called the "King of Drugs". The birthday of the "King of Drugs" is by legend the 28th day of the fourth lunar month and widely celebrated in memory of this medical genius.

Doctor Zhang Zhongjing and the Shang Han Lun

During the period of the *Han* Dynasty (circa 220 A.D.), *Zhang Zhongjing* (born with the name *Zhang Qi*) practiced medicine. This was some 240 years after the Warring States period (403-221B.C.). *Zhang Zhongjing* was dealing with a huge and deadly epidemic (believed to be typhoid fever) and he watched masses of people dying all around him. Over two hundred of his own relatives, about two thirds of his relations, had fallen ill and died from a plague in the area of *Jinjiou*. His determination and drive to understand and overcome disease must have been tremendous.

Doctor *Zhang Zhongjing* observed that acute disease was similar to an entire life cycle compressed into a very short period. From the onset of the disease to the end of life this life cycle could be divided into six individual stages each with its own unique conformation. The conformations for each of the various stages depend not only of the etiology of the disease but also the overall constitution of the individual and how the body is dealing with the disease at any given time.

When *Zhang Zhongjing* wrote about his observations of the six stages of disease, an acute disease called *"Shang han"* (which is believed to be perhaps typhoid fever) was common. *Zhang* made detailed observations on the progression of the illness and created suitable formulas for each stage. For each of the various stages, the *Shang Han Lun* provides a group of appropriate formulas, but the conformation determines the choice of the formula. *Shang Han Lun* applies not only to acute diseases, however, for its principles can be used for almost any disease situation as shown in the Japanese *kanpo* system used today.

Chart 2 (Typhoid Fever, fever progression)

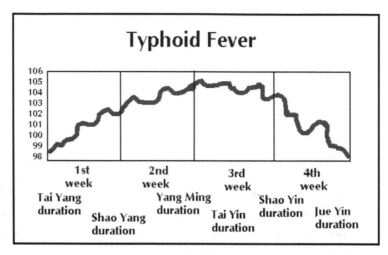

From observation one can recognize and determine the conformation, prescribe a matching formula, and cure the disease. Homeopathy resembles this approach in that the constitution of the patient and the main conformation determine the course of treatment.

From his devotion to combating illness came two of the greatest medical classics in Chinese history, *Shang Han Lun* and *Jen Kuei Yao Lue*. The *Shang Han Lun* (Book of Fever and Chills) deals with infectious, contagious, and epidemic fevers. While the *Jen Kuei Yao Lue* (Prescriptions from the Golden Chamber) deals with diseases that relate to digestive, respiratory, urological, nervous systems disorders, metabolism, gynecology, and other disorders. It is no wonder that *Zhang Zhongjing* has been revered as a medical saint.

Shang Han Lun and Japanese Kanpo

A brief history of the spread of Chinese medicine here helps to demonstrate the importance the classical "Old School Formulas" *Shang Han Lun* and *Jen Kuei Yao Lue*. According to Dr. Hong-yen Hsu, *"No matter how advanced a practitioner becomes in Chinese medicine, there, will always be a need to study the Shang Hun Lun and Jen Kuei Yao Lue and Six Stages relationship to disease."* Out of all the herbal information imported into other countries from China, none have been more studied and revered than these two medical classics.

There are 113 herbal formulas recorded in the *Shang Han Lun* and 110 herbal formulas recorded in the *Jen Kuei Yao Lue* written by *Zhang Zhongjing* of the *Han* Dynasty. The formulas from these two classics are known as "old school" formulas.

During the *Tang* dynasty over 6,000 herbal formulas were recorded in the *Wai tai mi yao* (Medical Secrets of an Official), compiled by *Wang Tao*. During the *Sung* dynasty over 30,000 herbal formulas were recorded in the *Tai Ping Sheng Hui Fang* (*Taiping* Scared Remedies), compiled by *Wang Huiyin*. The Pu *Ji Fang* (Prescriptions for Medical Relief) was written by *Teng Hong* of the *Ming* dynasty, who recorded over 61,739 herbal formulas. These prescriptions together with formulas from other medical resources now number well over 100,000. It is easy to see that the wealth of herbal knowledge in China goes beyond comprehension.

Chinese herbal medicine was brought into Korea during the early part of the era known as the "Three Countries"-- *Kokuryo, Baikje*, and *Shilla* (circa 300 A.D.). Herbal formulas from the *Chin, Sui*, and *Tang* dynasties were introduced in Japan from Korea in 414 to 700 along with other aspects of Korean culture. In the year 754 a celebrated Chinese Buddhist monk set up a clinic in Japan that provided free medical services, an event that heralded the beginning of social Practice of medicine in Japan.

It is interesting to note that as traditional Chinese medicine expanded to other countries such as Korea, Japan, and Taiwan, out of all the works on herbal formulas, the *Shang Han Lun* and *Jen Kuei Yao Lue* are still among the most respected and researched texts in these countries today.

The resurrection of herbal medicine in Japan after the Second World War

The resurrection of herbal medicine in Japan after the Second World War according to Dr. *Domei Yakazu*, (born in Japan 1905, graduated

from the Tokyo Medical College and became the superintendent of
Onjito Clinic, Tokyo) is due to these four main reasons:

1. *"The forgotten herb medicine of Japan regained attention with the introduction
   from the U.S.A. the medical theories of mentality and physique, Hans Selve's
   book "Stress", and other ideas, which were derived from the same origin as herb
   medicine."*

2. *"After the War, countries like France, Germany, Russia, and etc. did research
   on acupuncture. Esteemed Japanese scholars were often surprised at being asked
   about herb medicine during their visits in Europe. Naturally this directed their
   attention to herb medicine again."*

3. *"An important reason is that people lost faith in chemical drugs for the side
   effects they produce."*

4. *"China, the place where herbal medicine originated, accomplished a great deal
   in revising and developing herbal medicine. After 1958, the country introduced
   surgical procedures that incorporate Oriental and Western medicine by using
   acupuncture anesthesia. As a result, herbal medicine, which had been in the
   disfavor of the U.S.A., now became something the U.S.A. now began to view
   differently. Added to this were the biochemical investigations and research of
   herbal medicine by NIH (National Institute of Health) from 1973, and the
   recognition of herbal medicine by WHO (World Health Organization) of the
   United Nations from 1975."* [3]

Dr. *Domei Yakazu* also has stated *"The revival of herbal medicine is not just
a passing interest. More significantly, it is a return to nature, a nostalgic feeling
that arises owing to a painful experience brought about by the harmfulness of
chemical drugs."* In 1950 the Japan Society for Oriental Medicine was
founded as a government organization to research the academics of
Oriental Herb Medicine. The members of this organization consist
mainly of medical doctors who practice *"Kanpo"* (traditional herbal
medicine).

---

[3]   "The Development of Chinese Herbal Medicine In Japan", by Domei
        Yakazu, Bulletin of The Oriental Healing Arts Institute of U.S.A. vol.
        4, no.6 1979

Although in the past The Japan Society for Oriental Medicine had twice been rejected in its applications for admittance as a member society under the Japan Medical Association, in 1975 the Association set aside a day for panel discussions on herbal medicine and acupuncture. This was an event marking the beginning of a new era for herbal medicine in Japan. In October the same year, when the international doctors' conference was held in Japan, the Japan Doctors Association made the effort in introducing the subject of herbal medicine research in Japan.

Japan's *"Kanpo"* (traditional herbalist) doctors have contributed greatly to the research and modern-day use of Oriental herbal medicine. The Chinese medical classics *Shang Han Lun* and *Jen Kuei Yao Lue* are the two main texts that have been studied. The research on the "Old School Formulas" by these Western trained *kanpo* practitioners is proving how important traditional herbal medicine is for today's medical problems.

Chapter Two

Basic Theoretical Concepts Related to Six Stages

Overview

The main emphasis in this section is to develop a greater understanding of basic Chinese medical theory as it relates to the "Six Stages of Disease ".

- Cause of disease
- Qi, water, and blood theory (Theory)
- Meridians and the six energetic layers
- Concept of conformations (*Zheng* theory)
- The three treasures (fundamental foundation for all facets of life)
- *San Jiao (*Three Warmers or Three Burners)
- The progression of disease from the surface of the body into the internal organs

The Cause of Disease

Cause of disease *(Bing yin)*, according to Chinese medical theory, is that which produces disease. There are three categories of etiological factors known as *San Yin*. They are exogenous, endogenous, and non-exo-endogenous classification of causes of disease.

Exogenous factors *(wai yin)* are etiological factors that originate outside the body. They refer mainly to the six excessive and untimely climatic influences as well as pestilential pathogens.

Endogenous factors *(nei yin)* are etiological factors that arise within the body. These occur mainly due to excessive emotional changes.

Non-exo-endogenous factors *(bu nei wai yin)* are etiological factors that are other than the exogenous and endogenous factors. They refer mainly to factors such as; improper diet, overwork, sexual overindulgence, trauma, and animal bites.

Pathogenic qi or evil qi *(xie qi)* are factors harmful to the body and capable of causing disease.

Exogenous pathogens *(wai xie)* are those pathogens that originate outside the body, which include the six excesses and various infectious factors.

External affection or external contraction *(wai gan)* is the catching or developing a disease caused by exogenous factors.

Chart 3 (Battle between Disease and the Body's Normal Qi)

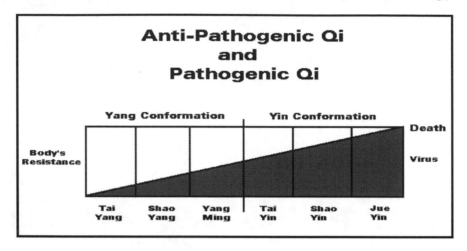

In Chart 2, starting from the left, the body's normal energy (anti-pathogenic qi) is strong and the invading disease or pathogen is weak. From the onset of the Taiyang stage to the Jueyin stage, if unchecked, the pathogenic qi will cause death.

Invasion of Pathogenic Qi into the Six Energetic Layers of the Body

All aspects and every cell of the body are influenced by *qi*. *Qi* (Life-force) circulates throughout the body by way of the *jinglo* (meridian) system to keep all in good order and health. There are different types of *Qi*. For example, *Wei qi* (protective energy) and *Ying qi* (nourishing energy) are the two main forms of *Qi* that circulate throughout the *jinglo* network. *Wei qi* is *yang* in nature, it is aggressive and fast, and controls the surface of the body by opening and closing the pores to help regulate heat through perspiration. *Ying qi* circulates within the meridians and is inseparable from blood and fluids as they nourish all systems of the body.

There are twelve main meridians or channels of energy that comprise the six energetic layers. Two meridians make up one energetic layer and two layers complete an energetic circuit around the body from top to bottom. Acupuncture points are located along these meridians, which act as gates or pathways connecting the surface of the body to the internal organs. It is via the meridian system (*jinglo*) and six energetic layers that pathogenic *qi* is able to travel around and attack the internal organs.

Chart 3 (Invasion of Pathogenic qi through the six layers)

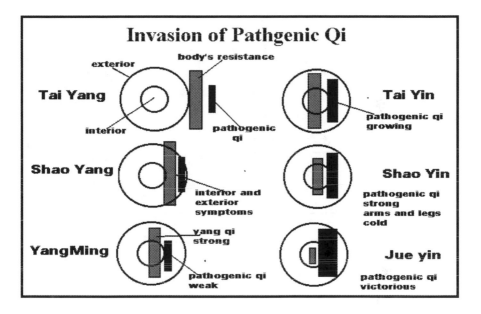

The Energetic Layers of the Body

The energetic layers of the body are the twelve main meridians of the body. These meridians are linked together at the fingers and toes to form large protective layers at the surface of the body. Their job is to keep the normal *qi* (energy) circulating throughout the whole system in order to protect and keep the body healthy and robust. Disorders within the energetic layers are considered surface or exterior conformation.

For example: Starting with the first point on the Hand-*taiyang* (small intestine meridian), SI-1 *(shaoze)* (located 0.1 unit (cun) from the ulnar corner fifth fingernail), we come to the last point SI-19 *(ting gong)* (located in a depression between the tragus and the mandibular joint). Here the flow of energy (*qi*) spreads out and deep into the head. When the *qi* surfaces again, it will become the Foot-*taiyang* (urinary bladder meridian) starting with UB-1 *(jingming)* (located in a depression 0.1 unit *(cun)* superior to the inner canthus). From here the *qi* follows the meridian down the back to the little toe to finish at UB-67 *(zhiyin)* (located 0.1 units (cun) from the ulnar corner fifth toenail). On the way down to the toes the *yang qi* is getting weaker and becoming more *yin* in nature.

The hands and feet are the changing points for the *yin/yang* relationship. The urinary bladder (*yang*) is connected to the kidney (*yin*), as the *qi* flow start back up the leg at the first point on the Foot-*shaoyin* (kidney meridian) K-1 *(yongquan)* (located at the sole and ball of the foot), the energy has become predominately *yin* in nature. By the time the *qi* has traveled to K-27*(shufu)* (located two units *(cun)* from the mid-line in the depression on the lower boarder of the clavicle); the *yin qi* is very strong. From here the *qi* flow goes deep into the body to surface again, at the first point on the Hand-*shaoyin* (heart meridian), Ht-1 *(jiquan)* (which is located at the center of the axilla). By the time the *qi* flow reaches Ht-9 *(shaochong)* (located 0.1 units (cun) from the radial corner fifth fingernail); the nature of *qi* has become more *yang* again. The heart (*yin*) and small intestine (*yang*) are connected at the little finger. This completes a full circuit of *qi* flow around and within the body.

Taiyang Jing energetic layer is composed of:

Hand-*taiyang* (small intestine meridian) and Foot-*taiyang* (urinary bladder meridian)

Shaoyin Jing energetic layer is composed of:

Foo- *shaoyin* (kidney meridian) and Hand-*shaoyin* (heart meridian)

    The *Taiyang* energetic layer and *Shaoyin* energetic layers complete one circuit.

Shaoyang Jing energetic layer is composed of:

Hand-*shaoyang* (*san jiao* meridian) and Foot-*shaoyang* (gall bladder meridian)

Jueyin energetic layer is composed of:

Foot-*jueyin* (liver meridian) and Hand-*jueyin* (pericardium meridian)

    The *Shaoyang* energetic layer and *Jueyin* energetic layers complete one circuit.

Yangming Jing energetic layer is composed of:

Hand-*yangming* (large intestine meridian) and Foot-*yangming* (stomach meridian)

Taiyin Jing energetic layer is composed of:

Foot-*taiyin* (spleen meridian) and Hand-*taiyin* (lung meridian)

    The *Yangming* energetic layer and *Taiyin* energetic layers complete one circuit.

One of the main functions of the energetic layers is to circulate the *Wei qi* (protective energy) so that the pathogenic *qi* is kept outside the body. It is through these meridian layers, that the exogenous *qi* or pathogenic *qi* works its way into the interior of the body and the internal organs.

When the anti-pathogenic *qi* of the body is able to contain the pathogenic *qi* at the surface skin layer or at the meridian and muscle layers it is called an exterior conformation. Once the pathogenic *qi* begins to affect the internal organs, such as heat in the intestines (causing constipation), it is called an internal conformation.

Initially, when the pathogenic *qi* invades the internal organs the response by the body is to produce a burning heat to destroy the pathogenic *qi*. This requires a tremendous amount of energy and soon depletes the body's qi and fluids. One of the first signs is a weak pulse and diarrhea, which signals a change from a *yang* stage conformation to a *yin* stage conformation. From this point on, strong, cold, and aggressive herbs must be used with caution.

The Concept of Conformations (Zheng)

A set of symptoms or syndrome related to a treatment is called *zheng* in Chinese medicine. *Zheng* may also be defined as a conformation, which can be a set of syndromes, symptoms complex, and or a treatment related to a specific disorder. When developing a diagnosis, it is important to consider all the various aspects of *zheng* for both the disease and the patient. Patients suffering from the same disease may have a different conformation due to different physiques and constitution: conversely, patients with different diseases but like conformations may take the same formula.

Each stage of disease has its own conformation or set of basic symptoms and a basic Treatment Concept. The same disease factor can have an acute or chronic conformation. People can have the same disease but different reactions depending on if they are young and energetic (strong conformation) or old and feeble (weak conformation). The same disease can progress to different levels within the same stage of disease. For example, a *Yangming* conformation can also have a *qi*, water, or blood conformation requiring different formulas that match the proper conformation.

An herbal formula can have its own conformation. Stiffness in the neck and shoulders is a Pueraria Combination (G*e gen tang)* conformation. "Major" formulas are usually related to a strong conformation such as Major Blue Dragon Combination *(Da qing long tang)* compared to a "minor" formula such as, Minor Blue Dragon Combination *(Xiao qing long tang)*, which is used for similar symptoms but a weaker conformation.

Six stages symptoms can have the conformation of being strong or weak. *Taiyang* symptoms with fever and no sweating (*taiyang* strong conformation) belong to a *ma huang* (ephedra) herb conformation.

Taiyang symptoms with fever and too much sweating (*taiyang* weak conformation) belong to a *Guizhi* (cinnamon) herb conformation.

Qi (Life Force) Jinye (Water), and Xue (Blood)

The theory of *Qi* (Life force), *Jinye* (water-body fluids), and *Xue* (blood) are very important concepts in Chinese medicine. In a healthy person each of these circulates freely throughout the body to nourish and protect against disease. *Qi* permeates into every cell of our body to promote their proper function. Body fluids and blood follow the course of the *Qi*-flow and are thus able to nourish and cleanse the whole system.

When disease invades the body and has affected only the *qi* aspect, the result is a fever to keep the pathogens away from the interior of the body. As the struggle between the protective energy *(we qi)* and the invading pathogen continue, the fluids of the body are used up and heat toxins begin to develop within the body affecting the blood. Therefore, the normal progression of disease may be seen as having an effect on the *qi* of the body first, then the water, and finally damage to the blood. Each of the six stages of disease also has a component of qi, water, and blood. There are however, cases when a disease starts at the interior aspect of the body and work its way to the surface such as in some cases of cancer.

Chart 4 (Qi, Water, and Blood Conformation)

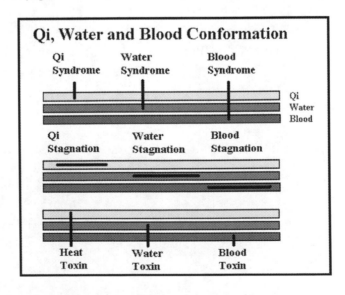

In the chart above there can be excess and deficiency within the qi, water, and blood levels. Stagnation may occur within any of these levels and may not have an effect on the other levels at first. As severe heat begins to damage areas of the body toxins will develop. Usually the progression of disease is from the *qi* level then water level and finally the blood level. Disease often will not follow the rules and therefore overlapping and erratic conformations develop. Knowing which of the six stages a disease has progressed should always be further refined to include the *qi*, water and blood concept. Using "*Qi* Formulas" for a blood conformation is like trying to catch a fish in the trees.

Qi Theory

Qi is the basic motive force of the universe that is seen as various dynamic functions and phenomena within all creation. *Qi* is the Life supporting energy flowing through all living things. It is the inner active force between *Yin* and *Yang.*

Dr. *Hong Yen Hsu* states that qi can be summarized as follows:

> *Qi theory: The origin of Life begins when yin and yang are unified to form Qi (Life force of all things). When the yin and yang are separated, Qi ceases to exist. Stagnation of qi can be the cause of all disease. Qi conformations can be divided into "mobile qi" and "static qi" according to a famous Japanese kanpo practitioner Dr. Keisetsu Otsuka. Mobile qi conformation refers to the up rushing of qi that causes dizziness, headache, vertigo, palpitations, flushing, and cold limbs. Static qi conformation means that the qi in the body has become obstructed and accumulated in one place. Stagnation of qi can cause pain and mental illness. The three main herbal formulas for this type of a qi related conformation are Pinellia and Magnolia Combination (Ban xia hou pu tang), Cinnamon Combination (Gui zhi tang), and Atractylodes and Hoelen Combination (Ling gui shu gan tang).* [4]

Jinye (Water) Theory

Jinye (body fluids), relate to disturbances in water metabolism, an imbalance in circulation, and or abnormal distribution of water throughout the body, which can cause a wide range of diseases. The terms phlegm, mucus, and sputum all refer to *Jinye* 'water conformation'. *Jin* (thin fluids), have the function of warming and nourishing the muscles and moistening the skin. *Jin* is clear and watery and is mainly located at the subcutaneous and skin level. Sweat and urine are examples of *jin* fluids.

Ye (thick fluids), have the function of lubricating the joint cavities (synovial fluids). *Ye* also nourish and lubricate the brain (marrow) and the spinal cord as cerebral spinal fluid. *Ye* fluids are primarily found in the bowels, bones, viscera and brain. These fluids are turbid and

---

[4]　　Commonly Used Herb Formulas With Illustrations, by Hong-yen Hsu and Chau-shih Hsu, Oriental Healing Arts Institute 1980

viscous. The distribution and discharge of *Jinye* fluids involve the spleen, stomach, lungs, kidney, urinary bladder, small intestine, large intestine, and *san jiao* (triple warmer).

Four Types of Water Retention Conformation:

Tan yin (literally, sputum drink) refers to water retention in the stomach. Fluid stagnates in the stomach and the intestines and results in borborygmus. Stagnate fluid below the heart can cause palpitations. The fluid obstructs the *qi* circulation and the lung *qi* fails to descend resulting in cough.

Zhi yin (branch drink) is accumulation of phlegm and fluid in the hypochondrium and epigastrium (pleurisy). Cold invasion can result in edema and fluid stagnation in the chest and diaphragm. Fluid retention above the diaphragm creates a feeling of fullness of the chest, asthmatic cough, dyspnea, and inability to lie down.

Xuan yin means that there is phlegm and water retention in the chest. Fluid stagnates in the chest and hypocondrium causing distention, pain with cough and shortness of breath. This type of fluid retention can cause fullness in the epigastrium, below the heart, and turn into heat manifesting as fever and sweating.

Yi yin (over flow drink) refers to water retention in the subcutaneous tissues (nephritis). This type of fluid retention, results in generalized edema and swollen painful extremities. Dampness obstructs the pores, hence general pain and very little sweating.

Main symptoms and signs of water conformation are: Edema, arthritis, dizziness, a heavy sensation of the head, tinnitus, palpitations, diarrhea, frequent urination poor appetite, no thirst, fullness in the chest and epigastrium, and general lassitude.

The main herbal formulas used for water conformation are: Hoelen Five Combination (*Wu ling san*), Polyporus Combination (*Zhu ling tang*), Minor Blue Dragon Combination (*Xiao qing long tang*), Major Blue Dragon Combination (*Da qing long tang*), and Jujube Combination (*Shi zao tang*).

Xue (Blood) Theory

Origins of Blood
The Ling Shu Spiritual Pivot or Devine Axis states: *"The middle san jiao (triple warmer) takes in Qi extracts the sap from it and turns it into the red substance that is called blood."*

Food is swallowed and the essence is refined in the middle *san jiao* by the *Zong qi* (*qi* of the chest or essential *qi*) and becomes *Gu qi* (grain *qi*). The fluids are distilled and the essence is extracted. This is directed to the lungs to mix with *Qing qi* (clean air) and is transformed into blood. The blood then flows through the blood vessels and is known as *Ying qi* (nutrient *qi*). *Zong qi* is formed, by the blending of *Gu qi* and *Qing qi*, therefore a cycle is complete. Kidney *jing* (essence) produces marrow *Sui*, which then produces bone marrow *Gui sui*, this in turn is transformed into blood.

The vitality of blood is not complete until it is united with *Qing qi* in the lungs. *Ye* (thick body fluid) flows with the *ying qi* (nutritive energy), within the blood, and from the lungs are circulated throughout the body. *Qi xue* (literally qi blood) is a term used in Chinese medicine. *Qi* and blood cannot be separated in our bodies and so the two words are commonly used together. Blood is a thick liquid form of dense *qi*. Blood nourishes and moistens the whole body. In the *Su Wen (Essential Questions)* it is stated: *"The liver receives the blood so there is sight; the legs receive blood and then have the ability to walk; the hands receive blood and so have the ability to grip; the fingers receive blood and are able to grasp."*[5]

Disorders of Blood
There are three basic conformations for blood related disorders: blood deficiency, blood stagnation, and heat toxins in the blood.

Blood deficiency can be a result of blood loss or diminished blood production. Insufficient blood fails to properly nourish the head

---

[5]   Occidental Institute of Chinese Studies Alumni Association, "The *Nei Ching* (Chinese Medical Classics)", Miami, Florida, (1979)

causing dizziness, pale lips, and sallow complexion. Restlessness, palpitation, poor memory, and fearful anxiety are signs of heart blood deficiency. Costal pain, blurred vision, twitching of the muscles, and numbness of the limbs, scanty light colored menses are signs of liver blood deficiency. The tongue is pale and the pulse is thin and or weak. *Tang Kuei Four* Combination (*Si wu tang*), may be used for these types of conformations.

Blood stagnation in local areas manifests as swelling. When blood circulation is blocked there is pain. If this becomes serious, palpable masses can be felt. Bleeding or bruising may occur when the blood vessels can no longer withstand the pressure form blood stasis. Stagnate blood becomes dark and manifests as cyan-purple lips and tongue, dry skin and an unusually dark complexion. The pulse has a general quality of being thin and rough. Persica and Rhubarb Combination (*Tao he zheng qi tang*) may be used for these types of conformations.

Heat toxins in the blood can be a result of febrile and other epidemic diseases. Blood heat conformation has symptoms such as: hemoptysis, nosebleed, erythema, menorrhagia, delirium and mental confusion cause by febrile diseases. The tongue is dark red or crimson colored and the pulse rapid. Rhinoceros and Rehmannia Combination (*Xi jiao di huang tang*) may be used for this type of conformation. *Yu Xue*, (stagnant blood) is known as a blood conformation. Blood conformations occurs more often in women because of menstruation and child birth which can result in poor blood circulation and blood stasis within the body. In Japan a blood conformation is known as *"oketsu"*. Research in Japan in 1986 showed that *oketsu* was a major factor for the following disorders: Sterility in women (11.2%), ovarian dysfunction (21.9%), cold conformation (82.2%), climacteric dysfunction (35.4%), and blood stasis of the pelvis (86.5%).

Symptoms and signs of a blood conformation are localized blood, stagnant blood, dysfunction of the peripheral circulation, and viscous blood. There are seven major herbal formulas used in blood conformation: Tang kuei Four Combination (*Si wu tang*), Tang Kuei and Peony Combination (*Dang gui shao yao san*), Bupleurum and Peony Combination (*Jia wei xiao yao san*), Cinnamon and Hoelen Combination (*Gui zhi fu ling wan*), Rhubarb and Moutan Combination (*Da huang mu dan pi tang*), and Persica and Rhubarb Combination (*Tao he zheng qi tang*), and Rhinoceros and Rehmannia Combination (*Xi jiao di huang tang*).

Doctor *Domei Yakazu* of the Department of Pharmacology, Tokyo Medical College has summarized "Diseases Easily Caused by Extravagated Blood *(Oketsu)* as the following:

1. *Gynecological diseases: hysteria, vaginitis, climacteric disorder, uterine myoma, endometritis, menstrual aberration, leukorrhea, sterility, etc.*
2. *Hypertension, arteriosclerosis, cerebral hemorrhage and degeneration, valvular disease, etc.*
3. *Chronic digestive diseases: hyperacidity, pepticulcer, gastrocarcinoma, gastritis, appendicitis, chronic constipation, hemorrhoids, etc.*
4. *Dermal diseases: eczema, urticaria, lupus erythematous, allergies, etc.*
5. *Bronchitis*
6. *Neurosis: disorder of autonomous nerves, mental abnormality, etc.*
7. *Accompaniment of sciatica, lumbago, etc.*
8. *Liver diseases: cirrhosis, chronic hepatitis, etc.*
9. *Urological diseases.*
10. *Tubercular diseases.*
11. *Various infections and fevers.*
12. *Ophthalmological diseases.*
13. *Trauma due to wrestling*
14. *Weak pulse[6]*

---

[6]   Considerations of Oketsu (Stagnation of Disordered Blood)", by Domei Yakazu, Bulletin of The Oriental Healing Arts Institute OF U.S.A. vol. 1, No. 1 1976

The Three Treasures (San Bao)

Traditional Chinese medicine uses the terms *Jing* (Essence), *Qi* (Life Force), and *Shen* (Spirit) as a theoretical concept to explain the human physiological system. They are known as the "Three Treasures" and are believed to be the fundamental foundation for all facets of life.

Jing is pure essence and is the fundamental material that is the foundation of life. It is the primal substance from which a new life is made. *Jing* is passed down from the parents and is known as prenatal *jing* and is the origin of *shen* (spirit) of a human being. Sperm is called *"jing zi"* which means "the son's of essence". When the *jing* of the parents combine a child is formed the *qi* begins to move and circulate and the *shen* (spirit) of the individual grows. Prenatal *jing* carried over from the parents is called *yuan jing* or original essence. The basic function of *jing* is to activate transformations and control growth, development, and reproduction. Prenatal *jing* cannot sustain life by its self after birth. Postnatal *jing* is the essence acquired from food, drink and air. The body converts and refines the essence or postnatal *jing* into various types of *qi* for all the bodily functions. *Jing* is stored in the kidneys and bone marrow. From bone marrow the essence of *xue* (blood) is first formed.

Qi, generally speaking, is the intrinsic substance that makes up and flows through the cosmos. It is the power and force of all creation and manifests in many ways. On a cosmic level there is what the Chinese call, *"Tian qi"* (heavenly energy). *Tian qi* is the empowering force of all things that live and grow. One form of *tian qi* is simply the air we breathe. Through the process of digestion the essence of food and drink becomes *Gu qi* (grain energy) and is refined into *zhen qi* (true *qi*). There are two aspects of *zhen qi* known as *wei qi* (protective energy) and *ying* qi (nourishing energy). These are combined with air *tian* qi in the lungs so that *qi* and *xue* (blood) can circulate throughout the body.

Shen is the manifestation and expression of *qi* and *xue* (blood). When the *qi* and blood are free flowing and healthy, a clear and bright spirit (shen) is apparent to all. It is *shen* that vitalizes the body and consciousness, and provides the expression for our personality and emotions. Traditional Chinese medicine states that the vitality of spirit (*shen*) is influenced by the seven emotions—joy, anger, pensiveness, worry, sorrow, and fear. Prolonged excessive states of emotional upset can disturb *shen* and thus cause disease (an internal factor or conformation). *Shen* is the mental energy and spirit directed by *Yi* (intent of the mind). The Chinese believe that when *shen* is cultivated and developed the senses and feelings become keen, the mind will be more alert, and thinking will become clearer.

Location of Disease and the San Jiao (Triple Warmer)

The body is divided into three areas known as the *San Jiao* (three warmers or three burners). The upper *jiao* includes the head and chest areas, the middle *jiao* includes that area of the body between the diaphragm and the umbilicus, and the lower *jiao* is that part of the body below the umbilicus. Disease of external origin can attack one or more of these areas of the body and work its way into the internal organs.

The normal progression of disease and its relationship to the various *jiaos* can be expressed as follows:

1) *Taiyang* diseases, attacks mainly the upper jiao
2) *Shaoyang* diseases, mainly attack the upper and middle *jiaos*
3) *Yangming* diseases, attack the middle and lower *jiao*
4) *Taiyin* diseases mainly start in the middle *jiao*, effecting digestion and energy levels (spleen and lungs) resulting in deficient *qi* syndrome
5) *Shaoyin* diseases, mainly attack the upper and lower jiaos resulting in poor cardio-vascular circulation and poor water metabolism *(Jinye)* with the heart and kidneys primarily being effected
6) *Jueyin* diseases mainly attack the lower *jiao*, causing a separation of the proper functioning of the upper and lower parts *(san jiao)* of the body. This primarily affects the blood *(xue)* level that is ruled by the liver and pericardium.

Chart 5 (San Jiao Relationship to the Six Stages)

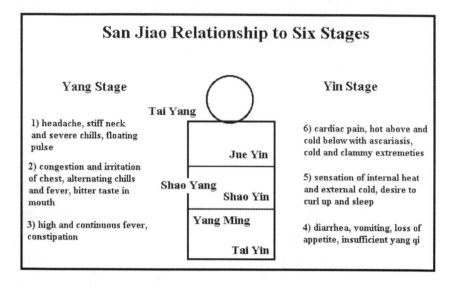

As long as the body is strong *(yang)*, and can produce enough heat to create fever, strong-cooling and aggressive herbs may be administered. When disease enters the *san jiao* levels while the system is weak and lacks heat *(yin* conformation), warming and toning herbs are generally used. During the *yang* stage, basically, disease travels form the head to the lower abdomen. If the exo-pathogenic factor is stronger, than what the *yang* of the body can handle, the *mingmen*-fire[7] will be damaged and diarrhea will result. These signals a change from a strong constitution to one that is weak *(yin)* and the internal organs are more at risk.

Treatment strategy for the *yin* stages is complex and not as clear as during the *yang* stages. Basically, during the *taiyin* stage the concept is to "tonify the center", *shaoyin* stage "strengthen the root" (kidneys), and for the *jueyin* stage "astringe and tonify *qi* while supporting and controlling blood".

---

[7]   *Mingmen* (Life gate or vital gate): this is the house of water and fire, related to the root of life. It is closely related to the kidney both physiologically and pathologically. The true fire in the life gate, life gate fire, refers to kidney fire, and true water in the life gate to kidney yin.

Proper evaluation of the location of disease within the body is very important. Herbs and formulas are designed to address various regions as well as the qi, water, and blood conformation associated with each part of the body. If a formula contains herbs that direct its effectiveness mainly to the interior and lower *jiao*, while the major conflict between the pathogenic *qi* and anti-pathogenic *qi* is taking place at the surface and upper *jiao*, it is similar to a general who sends his troops to the wrong battlefield to achieve victory.

External-Internal and Outer-Inner Relationships

In the theory of cold induced disease, exo-pathogenic *qi* or external disease factor starts to attack and invade at the surface of the body and work its way to the core. During the initial stage of disease, w*eiqi* (the most *yang* and outer defense of the body) meets the invading pathogenic force at the outer limits producing heat in order to destroy the pathogen. This stage of disease is usually acute, of sudden onset and short duration, with such signs as aversion to wind and cold, fever and chills, headache, stiffness in the shoulders, nasal congestion, sore throat, and a floating superficial pulse. This is known as an "External Conformation". External means the "body surface"; anatomically this includes the skin, subcutaneous layer, meridians, dermal vasculature, muscles, head, back, and extremities.

Internal means the inside of the body, indicating the circulatory and digestive systems or the internal organs. Internal disease may a raise from eventual penetration of external pathogens moving from the superficial layers to the interior of the body; from direct invasion of *zang fu* (internal organs): or from internal disharmony of the *zang fu*. Diseases with an internal conformation are more serious and chronic, of longer duration, and more gradual onset. Symptoms are high fever with no fear of wind or cold, changes in urine and stool, there may be vomiting, deeper pulse, and changes in the tongue body and or coating.

There is not a well-defined line that divides internal and external conformations. For those areas that are not clear the term "half internal and half external" may be used (usually relating to the *shaoyang* stage). Inner and outer also describe the disease location and supplements the terms external and internal. Internal means the digestive system, but also is used as a relative term. Inner indicates a wider concept. Outer is similar to external, but outer encompasses more than the skin and muscles intended by the term external. Both half external and half internal are "outer" compared to internal. Obviously, an outer conformation encompasses more than an external conformation.

In chapter I of the *Shang Han Lun*, symptoms of *taiyang* disease are floating pulse, headache, stiffness of the neck, and severe chills. These are known as surface symptoms. The basic "treatment concept" is to use formulas that cause sweating in order to clear the surface.

Dr. *Hosono Shiro*, president of the Japanese Society for Oriental Medicine in 1952 states:

"According to Shang Han Lun, a floating pulse, neck and shoulder stiffness and pain, and chills symptomatize the conformation. The floating pulse also known as a surface pulse is easily felt. Headache, neck stiffness, and chills of themselves are called taiyang disease. Whole body, joint, and back pain with shoulder stiffness make up a similar conformation. The common cold or initial stage of febrile illness often exhibit headache, neck stiffness, and chills with or without fever. If palpated, the pulse always feels floating, as in pneumonia, typhoid, or erysipelas as well as the common cold. Most every disease advance through this stage and depending on the duration of the illness or the strength of the patient's resistance may advance quickly or slowly. This resembles Hans Selyes' theory of the generalized adaptation response to disease. Zhang Zhongjing described the floating pulse as being of major importance. To diagnose taiyang disease, the pulse must be taken. Floating pulse, headache, shoulder and neck stiffness, and chill together delineate taiyang disease. The floating pulse alone cannot, as it may accompany other conditions. The principle symptoms of taiyang disease do not include fever because in the earliest stage of the illness, the patient has no sensation of heat. This is also known as the "wei level or stage of illness. Chills, however, are an important symptom of the taiyang illness."[8]

---

8   Shiro, "Ten Lectures on Chinese Herbal Medicine", Bulletin of the Oriental Healing Arts Institute of U.S.A. vol.9 no.3 May 1984 pg 120

Chapter Three

Symptoms and Treatment According to the Shang Han Lun

Overview

The main emphasis in this section examines the treatment concepts for the three *yang* and three *yin* stages of disease (symptoms and therapy) according to the Classic *Shang Han Lun*.

- Basic Treatment Concepts (Related to *Shang Han Lun*)
- Primary symptoms for each stage of disease
- Classification of herbal formulas used for each stage

Taiyang Disease Treatment Concept

Taiyang disease symptoms are a result of cold-wind invasion affecting the body at the surface layer. The *Shang Han Lun* states: *"The primary symptoms of taiyang disease are floating pulse, headache, stiffness of the neck, and severe chills. These are called exterior symptoms."* In *taiyang* disease, perspiration due to fever, mild chills and a slow pulse are termed *zhong feng*, a mild form of *taiyang* disease. A more severe type of *taiyang* disease with or without fever, is called *shang han* and is associated with severe chills, generalized aching, vomiting, hiccoughs, and a tense pulse when palpated deeply as well as superficially." The basic treatment concept is to use *"fa biao ji"* (sudorific formulas) to induce sweating and relieve the surface.

Shaoyang Disease Treatment Concept

In chapter three of the *Shang Han Lun, shaoyang* disease symptoms are described as a bitter taste in the mouth, dryness of the throat, and dizziness. Milder forms of *shaoyang* disease symptoms are impaired hearing, redness of the eyes, and congestion and irritation in the chest. The *Shang Han Lun* states: *"The primary symptoms of shaoyin disease are a feeble and small pulse and a tendency towards drowsiness. "*The basic treatment concept is to use *"he jie ji"* (harmonizing formulas). These formulas are used when there are half external-half internal symptoms and indicate that sudorific and purgative formulas are contraindicated.

Concerning the *shaoyang* stage of disease Dr. *Hosono Shiro* states:

> *"Alternating chills and fever indicate the expansion and contraction of heat. Chest distress indicates a heavy sensation of pressure from the chest to the costal margin. Objectively, palpation of the costal margin from the lateral to the medial aspect provides the key point in diagnosing shaoyang disease. The chest feels full, rather like the sensation that follows overeating. The quietness and lack of appetite reveal the patient to be too uncomfortable to eat. Irritability of the heart means chest discomfort with frequent dry heaves. These symptoms indicate a half external-half internal disease. The disease evil lies primarily in the chest and*

diaphragm affecting the liver. This area also reveals irregularities in circulation to the lungs. In addition, secondary congestion of hepatic circulation and the initial stage of liver function disorders may give rise to these symptoms."[9]

In relation to the three *jiaos* (triple warmer) of the body, when the disease is moving from the exterior of the body to the interior and from the upper *jiao* to the lower *jiao* there will be mixed symptoms and therefore the body must be harmonized at the *shaoyang* stage.

---

[9]   Shiro, "Ten Lectures on Chinese Herbal Medicine", Bulletin of the Oriental Healing Arts Institute of U.S.A. vol.9 no.5 July 1984 pg 256

Yangming Disease Treatment Concept

The *yangming* stage or sunlight stage of disease is a more serious condition than either *taiyang* or *shaoyang* stages. The *Shang Han Lun* describes *yangming* as occupying the internal region of the body and recommends purgatives as the treatment of choice for this stage. Symptoms are high and continuous fever, constipation, and strong abdominal fullness. *The Shang Han Lun states: "The primary symptoms of yangming disease are fullness and discomfort in the abdomen." "Taiyang disease treated with an [improper] sweating method may result in insufficient perspiration and change into yangming disease."*

A *yangming* conformation is called *"wei jia shih"* and is classified as either strong or weak. In a strong conformation, the disease evil (toxin) and contents of the digestive system combine to create a strong fullness (the abdomen is full and hard to the touch). In a weak conformation abdominal fullness is present but the abdomen is not strong (the abdomen is flaccid and soft to the touch). Strong purgatives should not be used for a weak *yangming* conformation. Instead formulas such as Gypsum Combination (*Bai hu tang*) should be used. Abdominal fullness is called *fu man*. There are two types, deficient fullness and excess fullness. In the deficient type there is fullness of the abdomen with no internal strength; in the excess type the abdomen is full with internal strength.

Taiyin Disease Treatment Concept

A weak digestive system and insufficient *yang qi* (functional energy) characterize the *taiyin* stage of disease. Symptoms of *taiyang* in the *Shang Han Lun* include abdominal congestion, vomiting, loss of appetite, severe diarrhea, occasional abdominal pain, and chest pain; therefore purgatives are administered. The *Shang Han Lun* states: *"The primary symptoms of taiyin disease (the inside disease of the three yin) are abdominal congestion, vomiting, loss of appetite, excessive diarrhea, and occasional aching in the abdomen. Stagnancy and hardness in the chest will occur if the case is treated by the purgation method (due to a mistaken diagnosis of stagnancy in the abdomen)."*

In *yangming* disease, abdominal fullness and pain with dry stools produce excess fullness and excess pain. By contrast, when deficient fullness (in *taiyin* disease) occurs, even emesis and diarrhea do not reduce the fullness. This is because the stomach and the intestines have insufficient *yang qi* and so purgatives should not be used.

Taiyin disorders occur in conjunction with a weak constitution and a functional weakness of the internal organs, so the patient easily contracts acute febrile diseases. A *taiyin* conformation is present not only in acute febrile diseases but may occur in other illness as well. *Shaoyin* and *jueyin* diseases have distal circulatory disturbances as part of their conformations and therefore exhibit cold extremities. The *Shang Han Lun* says, *"Shang han conditions with a floating and slow pulse and warm arms and legs indicate taiyin."*

Although *taiyin* disease exhibits an internal cold syndrome, it may be classified as either deficient or excess. If the tendency is towards weakness, formulas such as Ginseng and Ginger Combination (*Ren shen tang*) may be used. If the tendency is towards excess, then formulas such as Cinnamon and Peony Combination (*Gui zhi jia shao yao tang*) may be used.

Shaoyin Disease Treatment Concept

Weakened cardiovascular function and obstructed consciousness signal a basic *shaoyin* conformation. The *Shang Han Lun* says, *"The primary symptoms of shaoyin disease are a feeble, thin pulse, and a tendency towards drowsiness."* A feeble pulse means a very slight beat that may or may not be detected, as it is very weak. A thin pulse is like a thread, reflecting very weak cardiovascular function. Drowsiness means a lethargic state like sleepiness.

There are two differentiations for *shaoyin* conformation:

1) Whole body pain, earache, chills, sometimes fever, and the hands and feet are cold
2) Internal coldness with headache, diarrhea, anxiety, constipation, frequent urination, and clear white urine.

Jueyin Disease Treatment Concept

Cold and clammy extremities, cardiac pain and heat (irritability), and sinking, slow, and thin pulse are major signs of *jueyin* disease. The *Shang Han Lun* states: *"The cardinal symptoms of jueyin disease [a disease of yang within yin characterized by fever in the upper part of the body] are upward congestion towards the chest [taiyin disease is characterized by a downward congestion towards the abdomen], a sensation of hunger but no real desire for food, and vomiting of worms after ingestion of food. If the purgation method is used for treatment, prolonged diarrhea will result... jueyin disease is an imbalance between yin and yang which causes coldness of the limbs."*

The symptoms of *jueyin* diseases may be divided into two types:

1) Upper fever and lower chills (an uncoordinated condition of *yin* and *yang*, where the upper part of the body is feverish and the lower part is cold)
2) Mixed symptoms of fever and chills. "Mixed fever and chills" does not indicate the simultaneous presence of fever and chill, but rather that sometimes, fever appears and sometimes chill

appears. Occasionally these symptoms may be combined with the preceding symptoms of "*qi* flushing up", "fever together with pain in the heart", "hunger without desire to eat", "vomiting upon ingestion of food", and diarrhea with chills".

When upper body fever and lower chills occur simultaneously with a vomiting of ascarides (worms) upon ingestion of food, the main formula for treatment is Mume Combination (*Wu mei wan*). In a mixed fever and cold conformation, where fever and chill occur separately in the same bout of the disease the main formula to be used is Aconite and G. L. Combination (*Si ni tang*).

Jueyin diseases represent the utmost stage of *yin* diseases. In this stage, herbs for various *yang* and *yin* stages are used. Thus in Chinese herbal medicine, a *yin* disease is occasionally treated with a *yang* disease formula. The *Shang Han Lun* does not state that a *yin* disease need always be treated with a "hot" formula or a "tonic" formula.

Chapter Four
Combined and Overlapping Diseases

Overview

The main emphasis in this section is on the complications of combined and overlapping stages of disease that occur at the same time or not in the normal order and progression.

- *He bing* (Combined symptoms)
- *Bing bing* (Overlapping symptoms)
- *San yang bing bing* (Three yang disease overlapping symptoms)

Combined and Overlapping Diseases

Within the *yang* stages there may develop a combined or an overlapping of symptoms described in the *Shang Han Lun* as "*he bing*" (combined symptoms) or "*bing bing*" (overlapping symptoms). *He bing* is the combination of two or more stages of symptoms appearing at the same time. *Bing bing* develops, when symptoms of one stage quickly move into another and then coexist.

He Bing (Combined Symptoms)

When *taiyang-shaoyang* symptoms are combined it is called *[taiyang yu shaoyang he bing]*. The major symptoms are headache and fever *(taiyang* conformation) and bitterness in the mouth, dry throat, and dizziness *(shaoyang* conformation). When *taiyang-yangming* symptoms appear simultaneously, it is called [*taiyang yu yangming he bing*]. Major symptoms are headache and neck rigidity (*taiyang* conformation) and fever with thirst (*yangming* conformation). When *yangming-shaoyang* symptoms are combined it is called *[yangming yu shaoyang he bing]*. The major symptoms are fever and thirst (*yangming* conformation) and bitterness in the mouth, dry throat, and fullness in the chest *(shaoyang* conformation). When, three *yang* symptoms occur simultaneously it is known as *[san yang he bing]*. This is pathogenic heat moving from *taiyang* and *shaoyang* layers into the *yangming* causing symptoms of fever, perspiration, and abdominal distension, loss of appetite, incontinence, and delirium.

Bing Bing (Overlapping Symptoms)

In *bing bing* disease therapy, the general rule is "*xian biao hou li*". In other words, "cure the external first and then the internal." However, if the internal conformation is very serious or acute, it is treated first.

If at the onset of an illness two or three disease conformations occur in combination, this is described as "*he bing*" and the therapeutic approach is different from that of *bing bing*. The treatment method of *taiyang-shaoyang he bing* is to treat *shaoyang* first. If *"shaoyang-yangming he bing"* develop, then treat the *yangming* first. When all three of the yang stage symptoms appear at the same time, then whatever symptoms are the most severe indicate which stage is to be treated first. Sweating and purging methods should be avoided when *he bing* conditions develop. Instead "clearing heat" (dispersing heat) methods must be applied.

San Yang Bing Bing (Three Yang Disease Overlapping)

In *"San yang bing bing"* (three yang disease overlapping), even though the entire body feels hot, the heat has not penetrated enough to create a condition of excess in the stomach. Even though constipation may be present, the stools are not hard.

There is not a clear distinction between *bing bing* and *he bing* conditions; however, *bing bing* is generally an acute, excessive, and heavy conformation. *Bing bing* and *he bing* relationships only occur in the *yang* stages of disease. Similar relationships and overlapping of disease symptoms occur in the *yin* stages as well. These are called *"Jian bing"*. When overlapping of *yin* and *yang* symptoms occur it is still called *jian bing*. The rule of treatment is to treat the internal and external diseases at the same time.

The normal progression of disease from one stage to the next is known as *xun jing chuan*. The original order is *taiyang, yangming, shaoyang, taiyin, shaoyin*, and *jueyin*. Sometimes the progression jumps or skips one or more stages and is called *yue jing chuan*. There are times when disease moves from the exterior (*yang*) directly to the interior (*yin*) via the meridians. This is called *biao li chuan*, e.g., *taiyang* into *shaoyin*, *yangming* into *taiyin*, and *shaoyang* into *jueyin*. Exogenous pathogens can also directly attack the three *yin* meridians, by passing the *yang* layers and is known as *zhi zhong* or (direct attack). When the pathological condition of one or more meridians (stages) affect its respective internal organ it is called *fu zheng*.

Chapter Five

Conformations for the Six Stages

Overview

The main emphasis in this section is on differential diagnosis. A diagnosis is made from clinical symptoms and the understanding of the pathogenesis, in order to select the proper basic herbs and formulas for each stage. The patient's "basic constitution", is a factor that is often overlooked in making a proper diagnosis.

- Basic conformation for each "Stage"
- Main symptoms
- Pathogenesis (Causative factor)
- Differential diagnosis
- Therapeutic principle
- The patients constitutional factor (i.e. strong or weak body types)
- Charts for Differential Diagnosis
- Charts for Factors to Consider in Prescribing Formulas

Conformation for the Six Stages *(Bian Liu Jing Zheng)*

Diseases have their own unique functional pathology. In order to prescribe the correct herbal formula, it is important to understand not only the pathology of the individual disease but also the proper conformation and six stages relationship. A conformation is the basic symptom complex that each disease manifests within each individual. Conformation *(zheng)* is defined in Dr. *Hong-yen Hsu's* book <u>Natural Healing with Chinese Herbs</u> as:

> *"Zheng has two different meanings: Syndrome (set of symptoms) or a treatment. In modern diagnosis, the categorization of a disease is based on its nature and causative factors. In Chinese medicine, disease is also segregated by treatment. If, for example, it has been proven that a disease can be partially or totally cured with Ge gen tang Pueraria Combination then the disease is said to be the conformation of Ge gen tang Pueraria Combination. Patients suffering from the same disease may have a different conformation due to different physiques: conversely, patients with different diseases but like conformations may take the same formula."*

Each disease has its own unique "Six Stage" course by which it attacks the body. Disease and how the body responds to it must be closely observed in order to reveal the true nature of the pathogen and its treatment. The same disease or disorder may be treated with different herbal formulas depending on factors such as the original state (or constitution) of the individual as well as the disease conformation. Different diseases can be treated with the same formula if the six stages conformation is properly determined.

Yang Stage Conformations

Taiyang Syndrome (Taiyang Bing Zheng)

Main symptoms: Fear of cold or drafts, headache, neck and body ache, floating pulse, and fever

Pathogenesis: Wind cold invading the exterior

Differential diagnosis: <u>Exterior (meridian) excess syndrome</u> *(biao shi zheng)*, no sweating, fear of cold, and tight pulse; <u>Exterior (meridian) weak syndrome</u> *(baio xu zheng)*; sweating, fear of wind or draft, and soft pulse; <u>Interior (organ) symptoms</u> *(taiyang fu bing)*, the urinary bladder is attacked by the pathogen in an unrelieved taiyang meridian syndrome (taiyang jing zheng).

Therapeutic principle: Use spicy warm herbs for relieving the exterior, i.e., *ma huang* (ephedra), warms the body, causing the pores to open and perspire; while *gui zhi* (cinnamon) closes the pores, thus warming the interior of the body

Shaoyang Syndrome (Shaoyang Bing Zheng)

Main symptoms: Alternating chills and fever, distressing fullness of the chest and hypochondriac region, bitter taste in the mouth, dry throat, vomiting, and a bowstring pulse

Pathogenesis: disease is located midway between exterior and interior

Differential diagnosis: Exterior (meridian) symptoms, pain of the lumbar region and joints; interior (organ) symptoms, pain and fullness of the abdomen, and mild constipation

Therapeutic principle: Harmonize the interior and exterior

Yangming Bing Zheng (Yangming Syndrome)

Main symptoms: Feverish body with no fear of cold or draft; sweating, dislike heat, restlessness and thirst, and constipation

Pathogenesis: Excessive heat in the stomach and intestines

Differential diagnosis: Exterior (meridian) symptoms; high fever, profuse sweating, great thirst, and a flooding big pulse; organ symptoms (yangming fu bing), tidal fever, delirium, abdominal distention, resisting pressure, constipation, and a sinking firm pulse

Therapeutic principle:

1. Meridian symptoms; clear and disperse heat
2. Organ symptoms; attack and purge (herbs for this stage act fast (attack) on internal heat and quickly eliminate it)

Chart 5 (Yang Stage Conformations)

Stage	Symptoms	Pathogenesis	Differentiation	Principle
Taiyang	Fear of cold, body ache, fever, and floating pulse	Cold wind	Surface excess symptoms Surface weak symptoms	Relieve the surface
Shaoyang	Alternating chills and fever, fullness of chest, bitter taste in mouth, vomiting, and tight pulse	Disease located between surface and interior	More surface symptoms More interior symptoms	Harmonious relieving
Yangming	No fear of cold, feverish body, restless thirst, dislike heat, and sweating	Excess heat in stomach and intestine	Meridian symptoms Organ symptoms	Attack and purge

Chart 6 (Yang Stage Formulas)

Stage	Formula	*Yin-Yang* Relation	Patient Constitution	*Qi,* Water, Blood	Classification
Taiyang	Cinnamon C.	*Yin-Yang*	Weak	*Qi*	Sudorific
	Cinnamon and Peony C.	*Yin-yang*	Weak	*Qi*	Sudorific
	Ma-Huang C.	*Yang*	Strong	*Qi*	Sudorific
	Pueraria C.	*Yang*	Strong	*Qi*	Sudorific
	Minor Bupleurum C.	*Yang-Yin*	Strong-weak	*Qi*	Harmonizing
	Major Blue Dragon C.	*Yang*	Strong	Water	Sudorific
Yang ming	Minor Rhubarb C.	*Yin-Yang*	Strong to weak	*Qi*	Interior attacking
	Coptis and Rhubarb C.	*Yang*	Strong	*Qi*	Fire purging
	Major Rhubarb C.	*Yang*	Strong	*Qi*	Interior attacking
	Rhubarb and Mirabilitum C.	*Yang*	Strong	*Qi*-water	Interior attacking
	Melon Pedicle C.	*Yang*	Strong	Water	Emetic
	Persica and Rhubarb C.	*Yang*	Strong	Blood	Blood regulating

Shaoyang	Minor Bupleurum C.	*Yin-Yang*	Strong-weak	*Qi*-blood	Harmonizing
	Hoelen Five C.	*Yin-Yang*	Strong-weak	Water	Diuretic
	Pinellia C.	*Yang*	Weak-strong	*Qi*-water	Harmonizing
	Atractylodes and Hoelen C.	*Yin*	Weak	*Qi*-water	Diuretic
	Bupleurum and Cinnamon C.	*Yin-yang*	Weak	*Qi*-blood	Dual dissolving
	Bupleurum, Cinnamon, and Ginger C.	*Yin*	Weak	*Qi*-blood	Harmonizing
	Capillaris C.	*Yang*	Strong	Water- *qi*	Diuretic
	Polyporus C.	*Yang*	Strong	Water-*qi*	Diuretic
	Ma-Huang and Apricot C.	*Yang*	Strong	*Qi*	Sudorific
	Major Bupleurum C,	*Yang*	Strong	Qi	Dual dissolving
	Bupleurum and Dragon Bone C.	*Yin*	Weak	*Qi*	Sedative
	Atractylodes C.	*Yin*	Weak	*Qi*-water	Diuretic

Yin Stage Conformations

Taiyin Syndrome (Taiyin Bing Zheng)

Main symptoms: Abdominal distention with pain, vomiting, diarrhea, anorexia, soft and weak pulse

Pathogenesis: deficient cold (deficient yang) of the spleen and stomach

Differential diagnosis: Similar to *yangming* symptoms with overall signs of deficiency and a weak conformation

Therapeutic principle: Warm the center and strengthen Spleen

Shaoyin Syndrome (Shaoyin Bing Zheng)

Main symptoms: Deficient cold (deficient *yang*) syndrome; fear of cold, lying in a curled position, extreme cold limbs, weak and thready pulse; diarrhea, and fleeing of *yang*; Deficiency heat (yin deficiency) syndrome; restless insomnia, dry throat, dry mouth, and rapid and thready pulse

Pathogenesis: Deficiency and degeneration of the heart and kidneys

Differential diagnosis: Usually deficient cold but may result in deficient heat

Therapeutic principle: Restore the *yang*, moisten and clear heat for symptoms of deficient heat

Jueyin Syndrome (Jueyin Bing Zheng)

Main symptoms: Heat in the upper part of the body and cold in the lower part *(shang re xia han zheng)*; polydipsia, rising of yang qi affecting the heart, pain and heat in the pericardial region, hunger but no desire to eat, vomiting ascarides and extremely cold extremities

Pathogenesis: Internal deficiency with complications of mixed hot and cold symptoms

Differential diagnosis: Evaluation is determined on the severity of hot and cold symptoms

Therapeutic principle: Warm and clear (disperse) simultaneously

Chart 7 (Yin Stage Conformations)

Stage	Symptoms	Pathogenesis	Differentiation	Principle
Taiyin	Diarrhea, anorexia, abdominal distention with pain, and vomiting	Deficient cold in the spleen and stomach	Weak conformation with overall deficient *yangming* symptoms	Warm center and strengthen spleen
Shao yin	1) Deficient cold: fear of cold, lying in a curled position, extreme cold limbs, weak and thready pulse 2) Deficient heat: restless insomnia, dry throat, dry mouth, rapid and thready pulse	Deficiency and degeneration of heart and kidneys	Deficient cold, Deficient heat	Restore *yang*, moisten and clear heat
Jueyin	Heat in upper part of the body and cold in the lower, pain and heat in the pericardial region, hunger but no desire to eat, vomiting ascarides, and extremely cold extremities	Internal deficiency with of complications of mixed hot and cold	Evaluation is determined on severity hot and cold	Warm and clear simultaneously

Chart 8 (Yin Stage Formulas)

Stage	Formula	Yin-Yang Relation	Patient Constitution	Qi, Water, and Blood	Classification
Taiyin	Cinnamon and Peony C.	*Yin*	Weak	*Qi*-blood	Sudorific
	Minor Cinnamon and Peony C.	*Yin*	Weak	*Qi*-blood	Chill-dispelling
	Major Zanthoxlum C.	*Yin*	Weak	*Qi*-water	Chill-dispelling
Shaoyin	Ma-Huang and Asarum C.	*Yang*	Weak	*Qi*-blood	Sudorific
	Minor Pinellia and Hoelen C.	*Yin*	Weak	Water	Diuretic
	Vitality C.	*Yin*	Weak	Water-*qi*	Chill-dispelling
	Pinellia, Ginseng, and Mel C.	*Yin*	Weak	*Qi*-water	Digestive
Jueyin	Aconite, Ginger and Licorice C.	*Yin*	Weak	*Qi*	Chill-dispelling
	Licorice, Aconite, and Ginger Pulse C.	*Yin*	Weak	*Qi*	Chill-dispelling
	Mume C.	*Yin*	Weak	Qi	Chill-dispelling

Chapter Six

Traditional Classification of Formulas

Overview

The main emphasis in this section is on the twenty-four major classifications of herbal formulas used today. A general outline for each classification is given, followed by a list of related formulas, found within this book.

- General symptoms and indications for each category or classification
- List of formulas (from this book) for each Classification
- Contraindications and Precautions

Traditional Classification of Formulas

There are twenty-four major classifications of herbal formulas used today. In general, practitioners of Chinese medicine still use the classification system of *I fang qi chi* (a collective annotation of medical prescriptions) by *Wang Ang* of the *Ching* dynasty with three additional classifications added, *suan jiao ji* (smelling salts), *zhen jing ji* (sedatives), and *dou ma ji* (pox and measles formulas).

Once a diagnosis is made for any given disorder a treatment plan is developed and a course of action is taken. Knowing the basic classification of formula treatment strategies is the first steps in deciding what specific formula is best for the problem at hand. Making a proper diagnosis is similar to creating a masterful painting that is in harmony with itself. Before specific details are added the general scheme must be well defined. Here the general classification or "Treatment Concept" will help guide the practitioner to the appropriate formula for the individual conformation.

Keeping in mind the "Big Picture" of what we are trying to achieve is very important. It is easy to get lost in detail and not see the forest for the trees. The overall picture can become too cluttered. There is always a general "Big picture" to keep in mind when choosing the correct therapy: Does the patient need to be tonified, is there too much cold, is there disharmony at the blood level, or is the water balance off? These are basic types of questions that, when answered, will help define what class of formula to choose.

Combining the six stages theory with the general classification of herbal treatment helps to develop a more complete picture of diagnosis and treatment. Chinese medical theory uses the concept that: One formula can treat many different kinds of disease and each disease can be treated with different formulas. It is important, however, to use the correct formula classification.

Anthelmintic Formulas (Qu Chong Ji)

Qu chong ji formulas dispel or kill parasitic worms in the alimentary tract. Symptoms are a swollen and aching belly; loss of appetite or excessive appetite with craving for peculiar foods; and irregular bowel movements. The patient may become withered and yellow and emaciated. There are four classifications for anthelmintic: ascarides (kills nematodes), taeniacide (kills tape worms), oxyuricide (kills pinworms), and ankylostomiacide (kills hookworms). Proper diagnosis must be made before administering a correct formula.

Formulas in this book:

1. Ginseng and Zanthoxylum Combination *(Li Zhong An Hui Tang)*
2. Mume Formula *(Wu mei wan)*
3. Picrorrhiza and Mume Combination *(Lian mei an hui tang)*

Aromatic Inhalant Formulas (Kai Qiao Tong Guan Ji)

Kai Qiao Tong Guan Ji formulas are composed primarily of aromatic and "penetrative herbs" are used to treat unconsciousness or coma due to either heat or "chill closure". *Kai qiao tong guan ji* formulas are divided into, cool-opening or warm-opening. Cool-opening formulas awaken the patient and dissolve turbidity by means of the strong fragrance of the herbs. Unconscious patients with toneless hands, incontinence, feeble and minute respiration, and spontaneous perspiration cannot be treated with this type of formula.

Astringent Formulas (Shou Se Ji)

Shou Se Ji formulas are composed mainly of astringing and restraining compounds. They treat weight loss, physical debility and wasting, and exhaustion of *qi*, blood, and sperm. These formulas treat spontaneous sweating, cough, excessive menstrual flow, leukorrhea, spermatorrhea, uterine discharge, and urinary incontinence. They tone the skin and muscles, and control prolapse, astringe the lungs and intestines, and stimulate sperm production.

Symptoms of fever with excessive sweating, asthmatic cough with thick sputum, diarrhea due to tainted food, and excess heat that cause spermatorrhea are contraindicated for *Shou se ji* formulas.

Formulas in this book:

- Kaolin and Oryza Combination *(Tao hua tang)*

Blood Regulating Formulas (Li Xie Ji)

There are several types of *Li xie ji* formulas that help circulation and treat various blood related disorders. They are divided into hematinic (increasing hemoglobin), hemostatic (to stop bleeding), blood cooling, and blood warming formulas.

Pathological changes can cause the blood to overflow or stagnate, resulting in various kinds of hemorrhage such as epistaxis, hematuria, or blood in the stools. It is common to have conditions that require a combination of various "blood herbs" and care must be taken to use the correct formula for a proper treatment. A strong fever may call for a hemostatic and blood cooling herbs at the same time. A patient with a weak cold conformation requires both a hemostatic formula and a *yang* (warming) or "blood warming" formula at the same time. Major and minor symptoms must be noted and addressed in order to make a correct prescription.

Formulas in this book:

1. Persica and Rhubarb Combination *(Tao he cheng qi tang)*
2. Cinnamon and Hoelen Formula *(Gui zhi fu ling wan)*
3. Rhubarb and Leech Combination *(Di dang tang)*
4. Tang-kuei and Gardenia Combination *(Wen qing yin)*

Carbuncle and Dermatitis Formulas (Yong Yang Ji)

Yong Yang Ji formulas are used to reduce fever, relieve toxins, decrease swelling, soften hardenings, and eliminate carbuncles and dermatitis caused by either internal or external factors. *Yong yang ji* formulas are essentially antidotal, antiphlogistic, and fever purging in nature, and act primarily by circulating and nourishing the blood.

Formulas form this book:

- Schizonepeta and Siler Combination *(Jing fang bai du san)*

Childhood Diseases or Pox and Measles Formulas (Dou Ma Ji)

Dou Ma Ji formulas are designed to treat a wide variety of childhood disease. Acrid and cool herbs are often used to help drive the toxins to the surface in order to speed maturation of eruptions in the case of measles. Contagious diseases such as measles and small pox should be reported to the proper authorities, as they are quarantined contagious type diseases.

Chill Dispelling Formulas (Qu Han Ji)

Qu Han Ji formulas are composed of warm or hot natured herbs, and are intended to dispel chills in the viscera. They treat interior chill caused by *yang* deficiency, external chills that have invaded the interior, and increase the *yang qi* (warm energy), which has been injured by the ingestion of inappropriate food or medication.

Fever that is lying dormant at the interior can cause chills and the stronger the fever the more severe the chills. This type of condition is contraindicated for *qu han ji* type formulas. This is known as true heat at the interior with false surface chills.

Formulas in this book:

1. Aconite Combination *(Fu zi tang)*
2. Cinnamon, Aconite, and Ginger Combination *(Gui zhi fu zi tang)*

3. Evodia Combination *(Wu zhu yu tang)*
4. Kaolin and Oryza Combination *(Tong mai si ni tang)*
5. Licorice and Ginger Combination *(Gan cao gan jiang tang)*
6. Major Zanthoxylum Combination *(Da jian zhong tang)*
7. Minor Cinnamon and Peony Combination *(Xiao jian zhong tang)*
8. Tang-kuei and Jujube Combination *(Dang gui si ni tang)*
9. Trichosanthes and Chih-shih Combination *(Gua lou zhi shi tang)*
10. Vitality Combination *(Zhen wu tang)*

Digestive Formulas (Xiao Dao Ji)

Xiao Dao Ji formulas aid digestion and dissolve congestion--conditions are due malfunctioning of the spleen and stomach, impeded circulation of qi causing obstruction and distention, and movable and non-movable tumors which have developed from accumulations of moisture, phlegm, food, and blood. Digestion formulas stimulate the circulation of *qi* and blood and restore normal functioning of the organs.

Emetic Formulas (Cui Tu Ji)

Cui Tu Ji formulas cause patients to vomit sputum, undigested food, and/or toxins lodged in the throat, chest, or stomach. These formulas should be used as a short term measure for acute disorders. They should be used with extreme caution in the elderly and debilitated, and during pregnancy.

Formulas in this book:

*   Melon Pedicle Formula *(Gua di san)*

Expectorant Formulas (Qu Tan Ji)

Qu Tan Ji formulas aid in the expulsion or elimination of excessive "water" (sputum, mucus, and saliva). Sputum and mucus can be classified as either wet, dry, hot, cold, or "windy" (moving around).

Excessive accumulation of fluids results in "water toxins" as a result of poor function of the spleen and secondarily the kidneys. Most *qu tan ji* formulas contain herbs that tonify the spleen and support the kidneys.

Mucus or saliva can agitate or block the trachea, causing cough and an increase of sputum. It is common to combine these formulas with a cough suppressant.

Exterior-Interior Attacking Formulas (Biao Li Shuang Jie Ji)

Biao Li Shuang Jie Ji formulas treat both surface and interior conformation at the same time, or have a dissolving action in the interior as well as on the exterior at the same time.

Formulas in this book:

1. Bupleurum and Cinnamon Combination *(Chai hu Gui zhi tang)*
2. Bupleurum and Rhubarb Combination *(Qing yi tang)*
3. Major Bupleurum Combination *(Da chai hu tang)*
4. Pueraria, Coptis, and Scute Combination *(Ge gen huang lian huang qin tang)*
5. Siler and Platycodon Formula *(Fang feng tong sheng san)*

Eye and Vision Improving Formulas (Ming Mu Ji)

Ming mu ji formulas are specifically used to treat ocular diseases. In Chinese medicine the eye is divided into five regions known as a *"lun"*. For example, the pupil is the water *lun* and the iris is the wind *lun*. Each *lun* area is related to an organ and meridian. Based on diagnostic findings formulas are selected that also benefit the related viscera and meridian, such as, liver supporting or kidney tonifying formulas. Chinese practitioners often use the methods of wind dispersing, fever reducing, fire purging, or toxin relieving to effectively treat eye disease.

Fire Purging Formulas (Qing Re Xie Huo Ji)

Qing Re Xie Huo Ji formulas are composed of cold or cool herbs which are used to treat fever or fire conformations. These formulas are used when a harmful toxin causes a fever. It is important to distinguish whether the condition is deficient or excessive in nature.

Formulas in this book:

1. Coptis and Scute Combination *(Huang lian jie du tang)*
2. Gentiana Combination *(Long dan xie gan tang)*
3. Coptis and Rhubarb Combination *(San huang xie xin tang)*
4. Ginseng and Gypsum Combination *(Bai hu jia ren shen tang)*
5. Gypsum Combination *(Bai hu tang)*
6. Gypsum, Coptis, and Scute Combination *(San huang shi gao tang)*
7. Phellodendron Combination *(Zi yin jiang huo tang)*

Gyneco-Obstetric Formulas (Jing Chan Ji)

There is a wide range of conditions treated with *Jing chan ji* formulas. They are specifically used to treat female disorders and are used to treat abnormal menstruation, leukorrhea, fertility disorders, and problems associated with pregnancy and childbirth.

Harmonizing Formulas (He Jie Ji)

He Jie Ji formulas eliminate toxins by either coordinating the liver and spleen, or the stomach and intestines. Harmonizing formulas should not be used to treat surface conformation. This may cause the condition to advance to a deeper level.

Formulas in this book:

1. Bamboo and Ginseng Combination *(Zhu ru wen dan tang)*
2. Bamboo and Hoelen Combination *(Wen dan tang)*
3. Bupleurum and Chih-shih Combination *(Si ni san)*

4. Bupleurum, Cinnamon, and Ginger Combination *(Chai hu gui zhi jiang tang)*
5. Bupleurum and Peony Combination *(Jia wei xiao yao san)*
6. Bupleurum and Tang Kuei Formula *(Xiao yao san)*
7. Coptis Combination *(Huang lien tang)*
8. Minor Bupleurum Combination *(Xiao chai hu tang)*
9. Peony and Licorice Combination *(Shao yao can cao tang)*
10. Pinellia Combination *(Ban xiao xie xin tang)*
11. Pinellia and Ginger Combination *(Sheng jiang xie xin tang)*
12. Pinellia and Licorice Combination *(Gan cao xie xin tang)*
13. Scute and Licorice Combination *(Huang qin tang)*

Interior Attacking Formulas (Gong Li Ji)

Gong Li Ji formulas attack firmness in the interior of the body, and are also called purgatives. Purgatives lubricate the intestines, promote movement in the bowl, eliminate congestion and stagnancy within the stomach and intestines, and decrease edematous swelling of the abdomen and chest. These formulas should not be used when there is an exterior conformation.

Formulas in this book:

1. Major Rhubarb Combination *(Da cheng qi tang)*
2. Minor Rhubarb Combination *(Xiao cheng qi tang)*
3. Rhubarb and Aconite Combination *(Da huang fu zi tang)*
4. Rhubarb, Ginger, and Croton Combination *(San wu bei ji wan)*
5. Rhubarb and Kan-sui Combination *(Da xian xiong tang)*
6. Rhubarb and Mirabilitum Combination *(Tiao wei cheng qi tang)*
7. Rhubarb and Moutan Combination *(Da huang mu dan pi tang)*

Moistening Formulas (Run Cao Ji)

Dehydration or a "dry conformation", require *Run Cao Ji* formulas containing nourishing and moistening kinds of herbs. A dry conformation is either external or internal and can be seen as warm or cool. External dryness occurs mainly in the autumn. Internal dryness is due to exhaustion and a lack of visceral fluids. A dry conformation is treated mainly with *Run cao ji* formulas that contain moistening and mildly dispersing herbs or moistening, sweet and cool herbs.

Acrid and aromatic herbs that can exhaust and dry up fluids as well as bitter and cold herbs that damage the *qi* are contraindicated for dry conformations.

Formulas in this book:

- Ophiopogon Combination *(Mai men dong tang)*

Moisture Dispelling or Diuretic Formulas (Li Shi Ji)

Li Shi Ji formulas regulate the body's fluids and treat water related disorders. Fluids have the nature of being either, cool and *yin*, hot and turbid, or sticky and poisonous. Fluids are divided into internal-water or external-water conformation. Internal water conformation is further differentiated by the location in the upper *jiao*, middle *jiao*, or lower *jiao*.

Body fluids are affected by fever toxins, which are generated by wind, chills, heat, and fever. Diuretics improve water circulation and excretion of fluids. *Qu shi ji* formulas are prescribed according to the condition and presence of edema, jaundice, diarrhea, or dysentery.

In diagnosing water conformations it is important to discern a "*yin* deficiency" or "fluid drying up" conformation for which a diuretic is contraindicated. Bitter and arid herbs tend to dry out fluids and should be used with extreme care. For example, post-illness edema due to spleen deficiency or lower leg edema in pregnant women, are conditions requiring diuresis. Strong diuretic formulas for such conditions must incorporate other types of herbs that will supplement and tonify the *yin* and protect *qi* as well.

Formulas in this book:

1. Atractylodes Combination *(Yue bi jia zhu tang)*
2. Capillaris Combination *(Yin chen hao tang)*
3. Capillaris and Hoelen Five Formula *(Yin chen wu ling san)*
4. Coix Combination *(Yi yi ren tang)*
5. Hoelen Five Herb Combination *(Wu Ling san)*
6. Ma-huang and Gypsum Combination *(Yue bi tang)*
7. Polyporus Combination *(Zhu ling tang)*

Qi Regulating Formulas (Li Qi Ji)

Li qi ji formulas balance *qi* and treat all types of *qi* related disorders. Depending on the nature of the disease, these formulas are used to nourish *qi*, move and guide the *Qi* in order to improve blood circulation, purge accumulated *qi* in the lower *jiao*, and expectorate stagnant *qi* in the upper *jiao*. For conditions requiring *qi* tonic herbs that are treated by mistake with "*qi* moving herbs" the patient will become weaker and have a sensation of emptiness. When a patient with stagnant *qi* symptoms is wrongly treated with *qi* tonic herbs the condition will become aggravated.

Formulas in this book:

- Trichosanthes, Barkeri, and Pinellia Combination *(Gua lou xie bai ban xia tang)*

Sedative Formulas (Zhen Jing Ji)

Zhen Jing Ji formulas have a sedative and tranquilizing effect, reduce pain, arrest spasms, and help quiet hysteria. *Zheng jing ji* formulas are divided into two major groups. The first contain heavy minerals or shells that calm hysteria and relax the mind. The second group is composed of herbs that nourish the heart, calm the mind, and support the liver. Those with a weak spleen and stomach should be careful to use formulas that contain heavy minerals. They should be used with caution and for only a short duration.

Formulas in this book:

1. Bupleurum Combination *(Yi gan san)*
2. Bupleurum and Dragon Bone Combination *(Chai hu jia long gu mu li tang)*
3. Cinnamon and Dragon Bone Combination *(Gui zhi jia long gu mu li tang)*
4. Zizyphus Combination *(Suan zao ren tang)*

Summer-Heat Dispelling Formulas (Qing Shu Ji)

Qing Shu Ji formulas expel summer toxins and treat summer diseases. They act mainly by dispelling summer toxins or feverish diseases that occur when the weather is humid and hot. Heat dispelling formulas always include herbs that dissolve moistness, disperse surface toxin, strengthen *qi*, and promote salivation.

Formulas in this book:

- Bamboo Leaves and Gypsum Combination *(Zhu ye shi gao tang)*

Surface Relieving Formulas (Fa Biao Ji)

Fa Biao Ji formulas promote sweating, relieve muscle tension, speed eruption in measles, and eliminate surface conformations. Sudorifics act by expelling toxins accumulated on the surface of the body (skin and hair) which have not yet penetrated the interior. The sweating method is utilized to expel such toxins.

Most of these formulas treat acute disorders. They contain herbs that are light and volatile in nature and tend to lose their effiency when exposed to too much heat. Sweating can be further encouraged by having the patient bundle up after taking the formula. Excessive sweating can injure the qi and fluids of the body.

Formulas in this book:

1. Bupleurum and Pueraria Combination *(Chai ge jie ji tang)*
2. Cinnamon Combination *(Gui zhi tang)*
3. Cinnamon Ma-huang Combination *(Gui zhi ma huang ge ban tang)*
4. Cinnamon, Magnolia, and Apricot Seed Combination *(Gui zhi jia hou pu xing ren tang)*
5. Cinnamon and Pueraria Combination *(Gui zhi jia ge gen tang or Xiao ge gen tang)*
6. Cyperus and Perilla Formula *(Xiang su san)*
7. Gypsum and Apricot Seed Combination *(Wu hu tang)*
8. Ma-huang Combination *(Ma huang tang)*
9. Ma-huang, Aconite, and Asarum Combination *(Ma huang fu zi xi xin tang)*
10. Ma-huang, Aconite, and Licorice Combination *(Ma huang fu zi gan cao tang)*

11. Ma-huang and Apricot Seed Combination *(Ma xing gan shi tang)*
12. Ma-huang and Asarum Combination *(Ma huang fu zi xi xin tang)*
13. Ma-huang and Atractylodes Combination *(Ma huang jia shu tang)*
14. Ma-huang and Coix Combination *(Ma xing yi gan tang)*
15. Ma-huang and Morus Formula *(Hua gai san)*
16. Major Blue Dragon Combination *(Da qing long tang)*
17. Minor Blue Dragon Combination *(Xiao qing long tang)*
18. Pueraria Combination *(Ge gen tang)*

Tonics and Replenishing or Supplementing Formulas (Bu Yi Ji)

Bu yi ji formulas nourish and supplement weakness and deficiencies of *qi*, blood, *yin,* and *yang*. This classification of herbal formulas is divided into four major groups, *bu qi* (*qi* tonics), *bu shi* (hematinics), *bu yin* (*yin* tonics), and *bu yang* (*yang* tonics).

Precaution must be taken in prescribing *bu yi ji* formulas however. At times, a false-weak conformation is wrongly seen as a strong conformation. The patient appears to show signs of weakness and surface chills when in fact there is a firm fever at the interior of the body. If tonics are used it will aggravate the condition. Patients who exhibit a surface conformation combined with internal weakness or those with a weak conformation and excess symptoms must be treated with great care.

Formulas in this book:

1. Ginseng and Astragalus Combination *(Bu zhong yi qi tang)*
2. Ginseng and Zizyphus Combination *(Tien wang bu xin dan)*
3. Six Major Herb Combination *(Liu jun zi tang)*
4. Tang-kuei and Ginseng Eight Combination *(Ba zheng tang)*

Wind Dispelling or Carminative Formulas (Qu Feng Ji)

"Wind disorders" are broad in scope and can be very complex and should be treated with the appropriate *Qu feng ji* formula. Wind related disease, can a raise from either external factors or internal factors. External-wind is caused by the six excessive pathogenic factors that invade the body and lodge in the meridians, muscles, ligaments and bones. This results in a wide range of disorders such as headache, muscle tremors, and arthritic conditions. Internal-wind related disease, develop from general weakness and deficiency in blood. Internal fever toxins that affect the circulation of *qi* and blood may also manifest as internal-wind.

External-wind symptoms are dispersed with acrid and arid herbs. These types of formulas must contain blood nourishing and *qi* activating herbs in order to control the drying effect. Internal-wind symptoms should not be treated with dispersing herbs. Herbs that cool, moisten, and lubricate area used instead. Strong moistening herbs however, must not be used in excess as they may damage the *yangming*-fire of the stomach.

Formulas form this book:

1. Cinnamon and Anemarrhena Combination *(Gui zhi shao yao zhi mu tang)*
2. Tang kuei and Arctium Formula *(Xiao feng san)*

Chapter Seven
Basic Herbs and Formulas for the Six Stages

Overview

The main emphasis in this section is on the use of the primary "individual herbs" for each stage and the most commonly used formulas related to the individual herbs.

- Basic primary herbs for each stage
- Therapeutic principles and conformation for commonly used formulas
- Basic treatment method for each conformation
- Differentiation for various conformations (i.e. deficient cold/deficient heat)
- Basic herbs and related formulas (Charts)

Major Single Herbs and Related Formulas for the Six Stages

Basic Herbs and Related Formulas (*Yang* Stage)

Taiyang Stage

Main herbs: Ephedra *(ma huang)*, cinnamon *(gui zhi)*, and pueraria *(ge gen)*

Therapeutic principle: Use exterior-relieving formulas (fa *biao ji*)

Commonly Used Formulas:

1. *Taiyang* Weak Conformation (*Taiyang* Symptoms with Perspiration): Cinnamon Combination *(Gui zhi tang)*, Minor Bupleurum Combination (*Xiao chai hu tang*), or Minor Blue Dragon Combination (*Xiao qing long tang*)
2. *Taiyang* Strong Conformation (*Taiyang* Symptoms without Perspiration): Ma huang Combination (*Ma huang tang*), Pueraria Combination *(Ge gen tang)*, Major Bupleurum Combination (*Da chai hu tang*), or Major Blue Dragon Combination *(Da qing long tang)*

Yangming Stage

Main herbs: Rhubarb (*da huang*) and gypsum (*shi gao*)

Therapeutic principle: Use emetic formulas (*cui tu ji*) or interior attacking formulas (purgatives) (*gong li ji*)

Commonly Used Formulas:

1. Inside Weak Conformation (*Li Xu Zheng):* Minor Rhubarb Combination *Xiao cheng qi tang*, or Rhubarb and Mirabilitum Combination *(Tiao wei cheng qi tang)*
2. Inside Strong Conformation (*Li Shi Zheng):* Melon Pedicle Combination *Gua di san*, Coptis and Rhubarb Combination *San*

huang xie xin tang, Major Rhubarb Combination (*Da cheng qi tang*), or Persica and Rhubarb Combination (*Tao he cheng qi tang*)

Shaoyang Stage

Main herbs: Bupleurum (*chai hu*), hoelen (*fu ling*), pinellia (*ban xia*)

Therapeutic principle: Use harmonizing formulas (he *jie ji*) and moisture-dispelling formulas (diuretics) (*li shi ji*)

Commonly Used Formulas:
Half-Exterior (Surface) and Half-Interior (Inside) Weak Conformation (*Ban Biao Ban Li Xu Zheng*):

1. Weak conformation (*Xu zheng):* Minor Bupleurum Combination (*Xiao chai hu tang)*, Pinellia Combination (*Ban xia xie xin tang)*, Bupleurum and Cinnamon Combination (*Chai hu gui zhi tang)*, Bupleurum, or Cinnamon, and Ginger Combination (*Chai hu gui zhi gan jiang tang)*
2. Frequent urination: Hoelen Five Combination *(Wu ling tang)*, Atractylodes and Hoelen Combination *(Ling gui shu gan tang)*

Half-Exterior (Surface) and Half-Interior (Inside) Strong Conformation (*Ban Biao Ban Li Shi Zheng*):

1. Strong conformation (*Shi zheng):* Major Bupleurum Combination *(Da chia hu tang)*, Bupleurum or Dragon Bone Combination (*Chai hu jia long gu mu li tang)*
2. Difficult urination: Capillaris Combination (*Yin chen hao tang)*, Polyporus Combination (*Zhu ling tang)*, Ma huang and Apricot Combination *(Ma xing gan shi tang)*, Hoelen Five Combination (*Wu ling tang)*, or Atractylodes Combination (*Yue bi jia shu tang)*

Chart 9 (Basic Herbs for Yang Stage)

Yang Stages

Stage	Basic Herbs	Treatment Method	Conformation	Formulas
Taiyang	Cinnamon *Guizhi* Ephedra *Mahuang* Pueraria *Gegen*	Sweating	Surface symptoms with sweating	Cinnamon C. Minor Bupleurum C. Minor Blue Dragon C.
			Surface symptoms with no sweating	Ma-huang C. Pueraria C. Major Bupleurum C. Major Blue Dragon C.
Yangming	Rhubarb *Dahuang* Gypsum *Shigao*	Emetic or purgative	Inside weak symptoms	Minor Rhubarb C. Rhubarb and Mirabilitum C.
			Inside strong symptoms	Melon Pedicle C. Coptis and Rhubarb C. Major Rhubarb C. Persica and Rhubarb C.
Shaoyang	Hoelen (Poria) *Fuling* Bupleurum *Chaihu* Pinellia *ban xia*	Harmonizing and diurectic	Half-surface and half-inside (weak) symptoms with frequent urination	Minor Bupleurum C. Hoelen Five C. Pinellia C. Atractylodes and Cinnamon C. Bupleurum and Cinnamon C. Bupleurum, Cinnamon, and Ginger C. Atractylodes and Hoelen C.
			Half-surface and half-inside (strong) symptoms with difficult urination	Capillaris C. Polyporus C. Ma-Huang and Apricot C. Major Bupleurum C. Hoelen Five C. Bupleurum and Dragon Bone C. Atractylodes C.

Basic Herbs and Related Formulas (*Yin* Stage)

Taiyin Stage

Main herbs: cinnamon *(gui zhi)*, peony *(shao yao)*, and pinellia *(ban xia)*

Therapeutic principle: Use mild and warming or mild emetic *(cui tu ji)* and purgatives *(gong li ji)*

Commonly Used Formulas:
Inside Weak Conformation *(Li Xu Zheng):*

1. Vomiting: Ginseng Rhizome Combination *(Shen lu yin)*
2. Diarrhea: Cinnamon and Peony Combination *(Gui zhi jia shao yao tang)*, Minor Cinnamon and Peony Combination *(Xiao jian zhong tang)*
3. Constipation: Cinnamon, Peony and Rhubarb Combination *(Gui zhi jia shao yao da huang tang)*
4. Paralytic Intestines: Major Zanthoxylum Combination *(Da jian zhong tang*

Shaoyin Stage

Main herbs: Pinellia *(ban xia)*, ginseng *(ren shen)*, ephedra *(ma huang)*, and aconite *(fu zhi)*

Therapeutic principle: Use sweating formulas *(fa biao ji)*, harmonizing formulas *(he jie ji)*, and diuretic formulas *(li shi ji)*

Commonly Used Formulas:
Exterior Conformation *(Biao Zheng):*

1. Spontaneous Sweating and Frequent Urination: Ma huang and Asarum Combination *(Ma huang fu zi xi xin tang)*, Minor Pinellia and Hoelen Combination *(Xiao ban xia jia fu ling tang)*, Vitality Combination *(Zhen wu tang)*
2. No Sweating with Frequent Urination: Pinellia, Ginseng, and Mel Combination *(Da ban xia tang)*

Half-Exterior (Surface) and Half-Interior (Inside) Conformation *(Biao Li Tong Zheng)*:

1. Frequent urination: Aconite, Ginger, and Licorice Combination *(Si ni tang)*
2. Difficult Urination: Licorice, Aconite, and Ginger Pulse Combination *(Tong mai si ni tang)*

Jueyin Stage

Main herbs: aconite *(fu zi)*, ginger *(gan jiang)*, asarum *(xi xin)*, and licorice *(gan cao)*, mume *(wu mei)*

Therapeutic principle: Use chill dispelling formulas *(qu han ji)* and anthelmtic formulas *(qu chong ji)*

Commonly Used Formulas:
Chill Conformation *(Han Zheng)*:

1. Cold Exterior with Hot Interior *(Biao Han Li Re Zheng)*: Gypsum Combination *(Bai hu tang)*
2. Cold Exterior and Cold Interior *(Biao Han Li Han Tong Bing)*: Aconite, Ginger, and Licorice Combination *(Si ni tang)*
3. Hot Exterior with Cold Interior *(Biao Re Li Han Zheng)*: Licorice, Aconite, and Ginger Pulse Combination *(Tong mai si ni tang)*
4. Anthelmtic Conformation: Mume Combination *(Wu mei wan)*, or Ginseng and Zanthoxylum Combination *(Li zhong an hui tang)*

Chart 10 (Basic Herbs for Yin Stage)

Yin Stage

Stage	Basic Herbs	Treatment Method	Conformation	Formulas
Taiyin	Cinnamon *Guizhi* Peony *Shaoyao* Pinellia *ban xia*	Mild-warming or mild emetic and purgative	Inside weak symptoms with diarrhea	Cinnamon and Peony C. Minor Cinnamon and Peony C.
			Inside weak symptoms with paralytic intestines	Major Zanthoxylum C.
			Inside weak symptoms with vomiting	Ginseng Rhizome C
Shaoyin	Pinellia *Banxia* Ginseng *ren shen* Ephedra *Ma huang* Aconite *Fu zhi*	Sweating and Harmonizing	Surface symptoms with spontaneous sweating or frequent urination	Ma huang and Asarum C. Minor Pinellia and Hoelen C. Vitality C.
			Surface symptoms with no sweating or frequent urination	Pinellia, Ginseng, and Mel C.
			Half-surface and half-inside symptoms with frequent urination	Aconite, Ginger, and Licorice C.
			Half-surface and half-inside symptoms with frequent urination	Licorice, Aconite, and Ginger Pulse C.
Jueyin	Aconite *Fuzi* Ginger *gan jiang* Asarum *xi xin* Licorice *gan cao* Mume *Wu mei*	Chill dispelling Anthelmetic	Cold exterior with cold interior	Licorice, Aconite, and Ginger C.
			Hot exterior with cold interior	Licorice, Aconite, and Ginger Pulse C.
			Cold exterior with hot interior	Gypsum C.
			Vomiting worms	Mume C. Ginseng and Zanthoxylum C.

Chapter Eight
Differential Diagnosis for the Six Stages Syndromes

(Liu Jing Bian Zheng)

Overview

The main emphasis in this section is on differential diagnosis for clinical symptoms related to the "six energetic layers" of the body. These syndromes are of a more modern TCM (Traditional Chinese Medicine) perspective. The acupuncture points offered here are just "core points" to be considered and are not intended to be a full treatment.

- TCM diagnosis
- Symptoms
- Treatment principle
- Root formulas
- Primary acupuncture points

Six-Meridian Syndrome Differentiation
(Liu Jing Bian Zheng)

Taiyang Syndrome (Taiyang Bing Zheng)

Symptoms: Headache, stiff neck, aversion to cold, body aches, perspiration, and floating-tight pulse

Treatment principle: Eliminate wind and cold, relieve exterior

Formula: Cinnamon Combination *(Gui zhi tang)*

Acu-points: Lu-7 *lieque*, LI-4 *Hegu,* UB-11 *Dachu,* UB-12 *Fengmen,* UB-62 *Shenmai,* Du-14 *Dazhui*

Exterior Excess Qi Stagnation
(Feng Han Biao Zheng)
Symptoms: Fever, headache, aversion to cold, general aching, asthma with no sweating, thin white tongue coating, and floating tense pulse

Treatment principle: Relieve the exterior with pungent warm herbs, and facilitate the flow of lung qi to relieve asthma

Formula: Ma-huang Combination *(Ma huang tang)*

Acu-points: Lu-6 *Kongzui*, Lu-7 *Lieque* UB-11 *Dachu*, UB-12 *Fengmen,* UB-13 *Feishu,* UB-64 *Jinggu*

Exterior Excess with Restricted Meridian Flow
(Biao Shi Zheng)
Symptoms: Headache, general aching, stiff neck and back, aversion to cold, fever with no sweating, and floating-tense pulse

Treatment principle: Induce sweating, relieve exterior; promote production of body fluid, and relax muscles and tendons

Formula: Pueraria Combination *(Ge gen tang)*

Acu-points: SJ -5 *Waiguan*, GB-41 *Zulingqi*, UB-11 *Dachu*, UB-12 *Fengmen*, Du-14 *Da zhui*, Du-16 *Fengfu*

Exterior Cold with Interior Fluid Retention
(Biao Han Yu Yin Zheng)
Symptoms: Generalized aching, no sweating, cough, asthma with profuse white frothy sputum, aversion to cold, fever, headache, retching, no thirst, tongue coating white slippery and moist, and floating wiry pulse

Treatment principle: Relieve exterior, warm and transform interior *yin*

Formula: Minor Blue Dragon Combination *(Xiao qing long tang)*

Acu-points: UB-12 *Fengmen*, UB-13 *Feishu*, UB-23 *Shenshu*, Sp-3 *Taibai*, St-40 *Fenglong*

Exterior Cold with Interior Heat
(Biao Han Li Re Zheng)
Symptoms: Fever with irritability, headache, general aching, restlessness with no sweating, aversion to cold, thirst, scanty urine, constipation, and floating tense pulse

Treatment principle: Relieve the exterior; dispel cold and clear internal heat

Formula: Major Blue Dragon Combination *(Da qing long tang)*

Acu-points: Lu-10 *Yuji*, K-6 *Zhaohai*, UB-63 *Jinmen*, Du-14 *Dazhui*, LI-4 *Hegu*, SJ-5 *Waiguan*

Exterior Qi Deficient
(Biao Xu Zheng)
Symptoms: Headache and fever, sweating, aversion to wind, nasal congestion, retching, and floating-slow pulse

Treatment principle: Induce sweating, dispel wind, and regulate the nutrient energy *(ying qi)* and defensive energy *(wei qi)*

Formula: Cinnamon Combination *(Gui zhi tang)*

Acu-points: GB-20 *Fengchi*, GB-21 *Jianjing*, UB-64 *Jinggu*, UB-62 *Shen ma*, SI-3 *Houx*,
St-36 *Zusanli*

Mild Exterior Qi Stagnation
(Feng Han Qi Zhi Zheng)
Symptoms: Flushed face, fever, aversion to cold, and a weak and slow pulse

Treatment principle: Relieve the exterior with pungent and warm herbs

Formula: Ma-huang, cinnamon, pueraria, and pinellia decoction *(Ma huang gui zhi ge ban tang)*

Acu-points: Lu-9 *Taiyuan*, UB-62 *Shenmai*, UB-64 *Jinggu*, SI-3 *Houxi*, LI-4 *Hegu*, K-4 *Dazhong*, K-7 *Fuliu*

Restricted Lung Qi
(Feng Han Xi Zheng)
Symptoms: Fever, chills, cough, asthma, sneezing, headache, sweating, aversion to wind, tongue has thin white coating, and floating tense pulse

Treatment principle: Induce sweating, dispel wind, regulate the nutrient *(ying qi)*, defensive *(wei qi)*, and relieve asthma

Formula: Cinnamon, Magnolia, and Apricot Seed Combination *(Gui zhi jia hou po xing zi tang)*

Acu-points: LI-4 *Hegu*, LI-5 *Yangxi*, Lu-10 *Yuji*, St-40 *Fenglong*, Extra point-*Dingchuan*

Restricted Meridian Circulation
(Feng Xi Biao Shu Zheng)
Symptoms: Headache, stiff back and neck, fever, sweating, aversion to wind, and floating-slow pulse

Treatment principle: Induce sweating, dispel wind; promote the production of body fluid, and relax muscles and tendons

Formula: Cinnamon and Pueraria Combination *(Gui zhi jia ge gen tang)*

Acu-points: GB-20 *Fengchi*, GB-21 *Jianjing*, SI-3 *Houxi*, UB-10 *Tianzhu*, UB-11 *Dachu*, UB-62 *Shenmai*, Du-8 *Jinsuo*, SJ-5 *Waiguan*, GB-41 *Zulingqi*

Combined and Transformed *Taiyang* Syndromes

Taiyang Syndromes *(He bing, Bing bing, and Jian bing)*

Blood Stasis in Lower Jiao
(Xue Yu Fu Tong) (Taiyang Yu Yangming He Bing)
Symptoms: Tense hard fullness in lower abdomen, fever, normal urination, mania, jaundice, dark purplish tongue with or without purplish spots, and deep minute pulse

Treatment principle: Remove the blood stasis

Formula: Persica and Rhubarb Combination *(Tao he cheng qi tang)*

Acu-points: Ren-4 *Guanyuan*, Ren-3 *Zhongji*, K-14 *Siman*, K-15 *Zhongzhu*, Liv-3 *Taichong*, Liv- 8 *Ququan*, LI-4 *Hegu*, SI-3 *Houxi*, Sp-6 *Sanyinjiao*, Bl-17 *Geshu*, UB-25 *Dachuangshu*

Deficient Zang Organ Qi with Cold Stagnation
(Li Xu Han Zheng) (Taiyang Yu Shaoyin Biao Li Chuan)
Symptoms: Pain and hard fullness in chest and abdomen, appetite normal, frequent diarrhea, white sticky tongue coat, and deep tense pulse

Treatment principle: Dissipate cold, warm the middle *jiao*, supplement *yang*, and resuscitation

Formula: Ginseng and Ginger Combination *(Li zhong wan)* or Aconite, Ginger, and Licorice Combination *(Si ni tang)*

Acu-points: Ren-4 *Guanyuan*, Ren-6 *Qihai*, K-3 *Taixi*, Liv-3 *Taochong*, UB-18 *Ganshu*, UB-23 *Shenshu*

Diarrhea Due to Heat
(Xie Xie Re) (Taiyang Yu Yangming)
Symptoms: Continuous diarrhea (yellow, turbid, sticky stool with strong odor), burning sensation in anus, scanty dark urine, asthma

(with sweating), red tongue with yellow coating, and rapid forceful pulse

Treatment principle: Clear heat and stop diarrhea, relieve exterior and interior

Formula: Pueraria, Coptis, and Scute Combination (*Ge gen huan lian huan qin tang*)

Acu-points: LI-4 *Hegu*, St-25 *Tianshu*, Sp-9 *Yinlingquan*, K-7 *Fuliu*, UB-13 *Feishu*, UB-28 *Pangguanshu*, St-40 *Fenglong*

Excess Cold in the Chest
(Han Jie Xiong) (Taiyang Yu Taiyin Jian Bing)
Symptoms: Pain and hard fullness in hypochondrium and below the heart, constipation, no fever, thirst, and restlessness, hypochondriac pain with rapid breathing after eating cold or raw food, whitish slippery coating on tongue, and deep and slow pulse

Treatment principle: Expel cold and damp, remove phlegm and damp

Formula: Rhubarb, Ginger, and Croton Combination *(San wu bei ji wan)*

Acu-points: Sp-4 *Gongsun*, P-6 *Neiguan*, SJ-6 *Zhigou*, UB-17 *Geshu*, UB-20 *Pishu*
UB-25 *Dachangshu*

Fluid Retention
(Yin Zheng) (Taiyang Yu Shaoyang He Bing)
Symptoms: Fever or mild fever with sweating, aversion to wind, severe thirst, vomiting upon intake of fluids, dysuria, abdominal spasms, and floating rapid pulse

Treatment principle: Promote *qi* transformation, control water, and relieve the exterior

Formula: Hoelen Five Formula *(Wu ling san)*

Acu-points: K-3 *Taixi*, SJ-3 *Zhongzhu*, GB-43 *Xiaxi*, UB-23 *Shenshu*, UB-28 *Pangguanshu*, UB-64 *Jinggu*

General Pain Due to Ying Qi (Nutritive Qi) Deficiency
(Ying Qi Xu Zheng)(Taiyang Yu Taiyin Jian Bing)
Symptoms: General pain after profuse sweating, pale tongue, and deep and slow pulse

Treatment principle: Tonify *qi*, harmonize *ying* and *wei*

Formula: <u>Cinnamon twig with apricot kernel decoction</u> *(Gui zhi jia xing tang)*

Acu-points: UB-27 *Xiachangshu*, UB-60 *Kunlun*, K-9 *Zhubin*, P-6 *Neiguan*, Sp-4 *Gongsun*, Ren-4 *Guangyuan*

Globus Due to Water and Food Stagnation
(Pi Yin Zhi Zheng) (Taiyang Yu Taiyin Jian Bing)
Symptoms: Sensation of a lump or hardness below the heart (*pi* syndrome), borborygmus, watery diarrhea, reduced food intake, vomiting, odorous breath, abdominal distension, slight fever, pale tongue with white thick greasy coat or white curdy coating, and wiry or slippery pulse

Treatment principle: Disperse Globus, and water, harmonize the stomach, and pacify counter flow

Formula: Pinellia and Ginger Combination *(Shen jiang xie xin tang)*

Acu-points: Ren-12 *Zhongwan*, UB-20 *Pishu*, St-36 *Zusanli*, St-43 *Xiangu*, Liv-3 *Taichong*, Per-6 *Neiguan*,

Globus Heat Syndrome
(Pi Re Zheng) (Taiyang Yu Shaoyang He Bing)
Symptoms: Sensation of a lump (*Pi* syndrome) or fullness below the heart (soft when pressed), irritation of the heart, thirst, flushed face, hematuria, insomnia, anxiety, and floating tense pulse

Treatment principle: Clear heat and disperse Globus

Formula: Rhubarb Combination *(Da huang huang lian xie xin tang)*

Acu-points: H-9 *Shaochong*, H-4 *Lingdao*, Ren-14 *Juque*, K-5 *Shuiquan*, Liv-3 *Taichong*

Globus with Mixed Heat and Cold
(Pi Re Han Zheng) (Taiyang Yu Shaoyang He Bing)
Symptoms: Sensation of a lump *(Pi* syndrome) or fullness below the heart, vomiting, borborygmus, diarrhea, watery stool, thirst (for only a little drink), thin yellow coating on tongue, and wiry or thready rapid pulse

Treatment principle: Clear heat, disperse globus, support the *yang* and harmonize the exterior

Formula: <u>Prepared aconite decoction to drain the epigastrium</u> *(Fu zi xie xin tang)*

Acu-points: H-7 *Shenmen*, K-3 *Taizi*, Ren-4 Guanyuan, Ren-6 *Qihai*, Ren-14 *Juque*, Liv-3 *Taichong*, Per-6 *Neiguan*

Heat in the Chest and Diaphragm
(Xie Re Zheng) (Taiyang Yu Shaoyang He Bing)
Symptoms: Low-grade fever, insomnia, dyspnea with sweating, retching, diarrhea, *pi* (globus) below heart, ruddy tongue with slightly yellow coating, and floating pulse in *guan* (middle) position

Treatment principle: Reduce heat form chest and diaphragm

Formula: Gardenia and Soja Combination *(Zhi zi shi tang)*

Acu-points: Du-14 *Dazhui*, Du-9 *Zhiyang*, P-6 *Neiguan*, St-40 *Fenglong*, K-9 *Zhubin*, Ren-17 *Tanzhong*

Heat Retention in the Lungs
(Fei Re Zheng) (Taiyang Yu Shaoyang He Bing)
Symptoms: Distention in the chest, asthma with sweating, red tongue with yellow coating, and rapid pulse

Treatment principle: Clear heat from lungs; relieve asthma

Formula: <u>Ephedra, apricot kernel, gypsum, and licorice decoction</u> *(Ma huang xing ren gan cao shi gao tang)*

Acu-points: Lu-5 *Chize*, Lu-7 *Lieque*, Lu-11 *Shaoshang*, LI-4 *Hegu*, Extra-*Dingchuan*, Du-14 *Dazhui*

Heart Qi and Yin Deficiency
(Xin Yin Xue Zheng) (Taiyang Yu Shaoyin Jian Bing)
Symptoms: Palpitation, shortness of breath, pale complexion, lassitude, pale tongue with little coating, and knotted or intermittent pulse

Treatment principle: Nourish *yin* and blood, free *yang* and restore the pulse

Formula: Baked Licorice Combination *(Zhi gan cao tang)*

Acu-points: Ht-5 *Tongli*, Ht-7 *Shenmen*, CV-14 *Juque*, St-36 *Zusanli*, UB-15 *Xinshu*, Sp-4 *Gongsun*, P-6 *Neiguan*

Major Accumulation of Qi and Fluid Stagnation in the Chest
(Da Jie Xiong Zheng) (Taiyang Yu Yangming He Bing)
Symptoms: Pain below the heart (which is hard as a stone when pressed), pain and fullness in epigastrium, constipation, dry mouth, evening tidal fever and light yellowish or dry-yellow coating on the tongue

Treatment principle: Clear heat and remove water

Formula: Rhubarb and *Kan-Sui* Combination *(Da xian xiong tang)*

Acu-points: SJ-6 *Zhigou*, GB-36 *Waiqui*, LI-6 *Pianli*, St-37, *Shangjuxu*, St-39 *Xiajuxu*

Minor Accumulation of Qi and Water Stagnation in the Chest
(Xiao Jie Xiong Zheng) (Taiyang Yu Shaoyang He Bing)
Symptoms Fullness and hardness below the heart (which is painful when pressed), yellowish tongue coating, and chest pain on coughing, and floating and slippery pulse

Treatment principle: Clear heat and dissolve phlegm, disperse accumulation

Formula: Minor Trichosanthes Combination *(Xiao xian xiong tang)*

Acu-points: Ren-14 *Jueque*, Ren-17 *Tanzhong*, LI-4 *Hegu*, St-40 *Fenglong*, UB-17 *Geshu*, UB-20 *Pishu*

Palpitation Due to Spleen Deficiency
(Xin Ji Pi Xue Zheng)(Taiyang Yu Shaoyin Jian Bing)
Symptoms: Palpitation with restlessness, shortness of breath, lassitude, white moist coating on tongue, and slow weak pulse

Treatment principle: Supplement spleen; harmonize *qi* and blood

Formula: Minor Cinnamon and Peony Combination *(Xiao jian zhong tang)*

Acu-points: Sp-3 *Taibai*, Sp-4 *Gongsun*, St-36, UB-14 *Jueyinshu*, UB-20 *Pishu*, P-7 *Daling*, P-6 *Neiguan*

Upper Body Heat with Inferior Cold
(Shang Re Xia Han Zheng) (Taiyang Yu Taiyin Jian Bing)
Symptoms: Heat in the chest and cold in the abdomen, abdominal cramps and pain, nausea, diarrhea, white-yellow and greasy coating on tongue

Treatment principle: Clear heat, warm middle-*jiao*

Formula: <u>Coptis decoction plus stephania</u> *(Huang lian tang fang)*

Acu-points: Du-9 *Zhiyang*, Du-14 *Dazhui*, UB-17 *Geshu*, UB-*21Weishu*, Sp-3 *Taibai*, St-25 *Tianshu*, St-42 *Chongyang*

Qi Stagnation Due to Spleen Deficiency
(Qi Pi Xu Zheng) (Taiyang Yu Taiyin Jian Bing)
Symptoms: Abdominal distension and fullness (relived by pressure and warmth), anorexia, weakness, lassitude, pale tongue with white thin coating, and deep slow pulse

Treatment principle: Warm the middle, tonify the spleen, and relieve fullness

Formula: Magnolia Five Combination *(Hou po, gan jiang, ban xia, gan cao, ren shen tang)*

Acu-points: Ren-6 *Qihai*, Ren-13 *Shanwan*, St-36 *Zusanli*, Sp-4 *Gongsun*, Sp-6 *Sanyinjiao*, K-16 *Huangshu*

Shaoyang Syndrome (Shaoyang Zheng)

Symptoms: Alternating chills and fever, bitter taste and fullness in the chest and hypochondrium, reluctances to speak and eat, irritation of the heart, nausea, dry mouth, vertigo, blurring of vision, white tongue coating, and wiry pulse

Treatment principle: Harmonize *shaoyang*

Formula: Minor Bupleurum Combination (*Xiao chai hu tang*)

Acu-points: GB-20 *(Feng chi)*, GB-40 *Qiuzu*, GB-41 *Zulinqi*, SJ-4 *Yangchi*, SJ-5 *Waiguan*, P-6 *Neiguan*, Liv-5 *Ligou*

Exterior and Interior Symptoms Combined with Deficiency and Excess
(Biao Li Xu Shi Zheng)
Symptoms: Restlessness, fullness and oppression in chest and hypochondrium, delirium, heavy sensation in the whole body, dysuria, tinnitus, insomnia, red tongue with a yellow coating, and wiry and rapid pulse

Treatment principle: Harmonize *shaoyang*; clear heat, and calm the mind

Formula: Bupleurum and Dragon Bone Combination (*Chai hu jia long gu mu li tang*)

Acu-points: Liv-3 *Taichong*, P-7 *Daling*, Sp-21 *Dabao*, LI-4 *Hegu*, SJ-5 *Waiguan*, GB-41 *Zulinqi*

Qi and Water Stagnation
(Shui Qi Zheng)
Symptoms: Fullness and oppression in chest and hypochondrium, alternating fever and chills, irritation of the heart, thirst, sweating only on head, dysuria, and tight pulse

Treatment principle: Harmonize *shaoyang*, warm and transform water accumulation

Formula: Bupleurum, Cinnamon, and Ginger Combination *(Chai hu gui zhi gan jian tang)*

Acu-points: GB-20 *Fengchi*, GB-40 *Qiuxu*, UB-23 *Shenshu*, Liv-5 *Ligou*, Liv-13 *Zhangmen)*

Combined *Shaoyang* Syndromes

Shaoyang Syndromes (He Bing and Bing Bing)

Shaoyang Combined with Yangming
(Shaoyang Yu Yangming He Bing)
Symptoms: Fullness in the chest and hypochondrium, alternating chills and fever, afternoon fever, retching, hard globus *(pi)* below the heart, constipation, dry yellow coating of the tongue, and a wiry and strong pulse

Treatment principle: Harmonize *shaoyang*, clear internal heat

Formula: Major Bupleurum Combination *(Da chai hu tang)*

Acu-points: GB-36 *Waiqiu*, GB-44 *Zuqiaoyin*, Liv-3 *Taichong*, Du-9 *Zhiyang*, SJ-6 *Zhigou*,

Shaoyang Combined with Exterior Syndrome
(Taiyang Yu Shaoyang He Bing)
Symptoms: Fever with slight chill, pain and congestion below the heart, severe pain in the extremities and joints, slight nausea, depression, and floating-tight pulse

Treatment principle: Harmonize *shaoyang*, relieve exterior and dispel cold wind

Formula: Bupleurum and Cinnamon Combination *(Chai hu gui zhi tang)*

Acu-points: SI-4 *Wangu*, UB-63 *Jinmen*, SJ-5 *Waiguan*, GB-41 *Zulinqi*

Yangming Syndrome (Yangming Bing Zheng)

Symptoms: High fever, profuse sweating, thirst, aversion to heat, excessive urination, and forceful and rapid pulse

Treatment principle: Clear heat from *yangming*

Formula: Gypsum Combination (*Bai hu tang*)

Acu-points: SJ-6 *Zhigou*, Liv-3 *Taichong*, LI-1 *Shangyang*, LI-4 *Hegu*, LI-11 *Quchi*, St-44 *Neiting*, St-45 *Lidui*

Abdominal Fullness due to Excessive Dryness
(Zao Qi Hua Re Zheng) (Yang Ming Bing Zheng)
Symptoms: Abdominal distension and fullness caused by the improper use of emetics, fever unabated by sweating, aversion to heat, delirium, dry mouth and tongue, deep and forceful pulse

Treatment principle: Remove heat, harmonize stomach, eliminate dryness, and soften the stool

Formula: Rhubarb and Mirabilitum Combination *(Tiao wei cheng qi tang)*

Acu-points: Ren-12 *Zhongwan*, St-25 *Tianshu*, St-44 *Neiting*, LI-4 *Hegu*, LI-11 *Quchi*,

Dry Stool Due to Yangming Fu Excess
(Yangming Fu Shi Zheng)
Symptoms: Tidal fever, delirium, constipation lasting for six to seven days, restlessness, slight fever, low spirit, blurring of vision, and abdominal fullness and pain after improper use of a diaphoretic, dry mouth and tongue, deep and excess pulse

Treatment principle: Eliminate excessive heat and remove dryness

Formula: Major Rhubarb Combination *(Da chang qi tang)*

Acu-points: SJ-6 *Zhigou*, St-25 *Tianshu*, St-37 *Shangjuxu*, St-45 *Lidui*, LI-1 *Shangyang*,
UB-25 *Dachangshu*

Excess Heat Injuring Body Fluids
(Li Re Yin Zheng)
Symptoms: Severe thirst, spontaneous sweating, aversion to heat, irritation of the heart, scanty and condensed urine, full rapid and taut pulse, and reddened tongue with yellow coating

Treatment principle: Clear heat and promote the production of body fluids

Formula: Ginseng and Gypsum Combination *(Bai hu jia ren shen tang)*

Acu-points: LI-1 *Shangyang*, LI-4 *Hegu*, Lu-11 *Shaoshang*, UB-21 *Weishu*, UB-63 *Jinmen*, St-36 *Zusanli*, St-44 *Neiting*

Fluid and Heat Intermingling (Damp-heat moving downward)
(Shi Re Xia Zhu Zheng)
Symptoms: Fever, thirst, dysuria, insomnia due to irritation, cough, vomiting, dysentery, turbid urine, red tongue with little coating, and floating pulse

Treatment principle: Nourish *yin* and remove water and heat

Formula: Polyporus Combination *(Zhu ling tang)*

Acu-points: Ren-3 *Yaoyangguan*, K-3 *Taixi*, K-5 *Shuiquan*, UB-28 *Pangguanshu*, Sp-6 *Sanyinjiao*, Liv-2 *Xingjian*

Heat Disturbing Chest and Diaphragm
(Yang Ming Bing Zheng)
Symptoms: Abdominal distention with dyspnea, heavy sensation in the body, dry mouth and throat, fever, sweating, burning sensation in

the heart, aversion to heat, restlessness and insomnia, ruddy tongue with slightly yellow coating, and rapid pulse

Treatment principle: Clear stagnant heat from chest and diaphragm

Formula: Gardenia and Soja Combination *(Zhi zi shi tang)*

Acu-points: S-21 *Liangmen,* St-44 *Neiting,* Du-9 *Zhiyang,* Du-14 *Dazhui,* K-9 *Zhubin,* Per-6 *Neiguan*

Stomach and Colon Dryness Damaging Fluids
(Zao Qi Hua Re Zheng) (Yang Ming Bing Zheng)
Symptoms: Hard stool, irritation of the heart, delirium, mild restlessness, frequent urination, and constipation caused by improper use of a diaphoretic, emetic or purgative, deep and strong or slippery pulse
Note: (Overall milder symptoms than for Rhubarb and Mirabilitum Combination)

Treatment principle: Remove heat, promote excretion, and eliminate stagnation and fullness

Formula: Minor Rhubarb Combination *(Xiao cheng qi tang)*

Acu-points: St-37 *Shangjuxu,* Lu-7 *Lieque,* K-6 *Zhaohai,* UB-25 *Dachangshu*

Yangming Fu Organ Excess
(Yangming Fu Shi Zheng)
Symptoms: Delirium, tidal fever, fullness and pain in abdomen, abdomen painful upon pressure, sweating over the hands and feet, hard stools, dry-yellow coating of the tongue, and deep forceful pulse

Treatment principle: Remove dryness

Formula: Third modification of rectify the qi powder *(San jia jian zheng qi san)*

Acu-points: St-25 *Tianshu*, St-37 *Shangjuxu*, St-45 *Lidui*, LI-1 *Shangyang*, SJ-6 *Zhigou*, UB-25 *Dachangshu*

Yangming Meridian Excess Heat
(Yangming Jing Shi Re Zheng)
Symptoms: High fever, profuse sweating, severe thirst, thin dry-yellow coating of the tongue, and full pulse

Treatment principle: Clear heat from *yangming* meridian

Formula: Gypsum Combination *(Bai hu tang)*

Acu-points: St-44 *Neitaing*, LI-11 *Quchi*, P-6 *Neiguan*, LI-4 *Hegu*

Yangming Meridian Syndrome
(Yangming Jing Bing Zheng)
Symptoms: Profuse sweating, high fever, thirst, and rolling, forceful, and full pulse

Treatment principle: Clear heat

Formula: Gypsum Combination *(Bai hu tang)*

Acu-points: LI-4 *Hegu*, LI-11 *Quchi*, St-44 *Neiting*, Liv-2 *Xingjian*

Yangming (He Bing and Bing Bing) Syndrome

Blood Stasis
(Xue Yu Fu Tong Zheng) (Yangming Yu Shaoyang He Bing)
Symptoms: Manic behavior, poor memory, black hard stool (easily defecated), dysuria, polyuria, thirst and dry mouth, distention in lower abdomen which is painful to press, constipation lasting for six to seven days, tongue red, and a firm and rapid pulse

Treatment principle: Remove blood stasis

Formula: Rhubarb and Leech Combination *(Di dang tang)*

Acu-points: Ren-4 *Guanyuan,* K-14 *Siman,* K-15 *Zhongzu,* Lu-9 *Taiyuan,* H-7 *Shenmen,* Du-20 *Baihui,* UB-27 *Xiaochangshu*

Jaundice
(Huang Dan Zheng) (Yangming Yu Shaoyang He Bing)
Symptoms: Jaundice skin and sclera, dark yellow and scanty urine, no sweating, dysuria, nausea, burning sensation in the region of the heart, dry mouth and throat, upper abdominal fullness, tongue red with sticky yellow coating, slippery and rapid pulse

Treatment principle: Clear damp heat and remove jaundice

Formula: Capillaris Combination *(Yin chen hao tang)*

Acu-points: St-37 *Shang juxu,* St-42 *Chongyang,* GB-34 *Yanglingquan,* SI-4 *Wangu,* P-7 *Daling,* SJ-5 *Waiguan,* UB-19 *Danshu*

Taiyin Bing Zheng Syndrome

Cold Stagnation
(Han Zheng) (Taiyin Bing Zheng)
Symptoms: a delicate constitution, abdominal pain, diarrhea, abdominal distention, and spasms in the abdomen, dry mouth and polyuria, pale tongue with white coating, and tight pulse

Treatment principle: Warm the middle *jiao* and relieve cold, strengthen spleen

Formula: Cinnamon and Peony Combination *(Gui zhi jia shao yao tang)*

Acu-points: Ren-12 *Zhongwan*, St-25 *Tianshu*, St-36 *Zusanli*, Sp-3 *Taibai*, Sp-9 *Yinlingquan*

Qi Deficiency with Cold Stagnation
(Qi Xu Han Zheng) (Taiyin Bing Zheng)
Symptoms: delicate constitution with a tendency towards fatigue, diarrhea, feverish sensation in the palms and soles, night sweats, pale tongue with white coating, and weak pulse

Treatment principle: Warm stomach and spleen, supplement deficiency

Formula: Minor Cinnamon and Peony Combination *(Xiao jian zhong tang)*

Acu-points: Ren-12 *Zhongwan*, UB-20 *Pishu*, UB-21 *Weishu*, St-36 *Zusanli*, Sp-3 *Taibai*

Taiyin Syndrome
(Taiyin Bing Zheng)
Symptoms: Intermittent abdominal (pain with preference to warmth and pressure), vomiting, diarrhea, anorexia, no thirst, pale tongue with white coating, and deep pulse

Treatment principle: Warm *yang* and remove cold

Formula: <u>Regulate the Middle Pill</u> *(Li zhong wan)*

Acu-points: Ren-12 *Zhongwan*, UB-20 *Pishu*, St-36 *Zusanli*, Sp-3 *Taibai*, Sp-9 *Yinlingquan*

Taiyin (Jian Bing) Syndrome

Cold Damp Stagnation
(Han Shi Zheng) (Taiyin Yu Shaoyang Jian Bing)
Symptoms: Dark yellowish skin (as if smoked), jaundice sclera, dark urine, no fever, pale tongue with white sticky coating, and deep slow pulse

Treatment principle: Warm the middle *jiao* and relieve cold, strengthen spleen, and eliminate damp

Formula: Capillaris and Hoelen Five Formula *(Yin chen wu ling san)*

Acu-points: Sp-4 *Gongsun,* Sp-9 *Yinlingquan,* SI-4 *Wangu*), Ren-12 *Zhongwan,* St-25 *Tianshu,* UB-18 *Ganshu,* UB-19 *Danshu, SJ-3 Zhongshu*

Taiyin Disease with Exterior Syndrome
(Taiyin Yu Taiyang Jian Bing Zheng)
Symptoms: *Taiyin* symptoms with a floating pulse; characterized by decline of spleen yang with production of cold damp in the interior

Treatment principle: Regulate the spleen and stomach, and harmonize *ying* (nutritive *qi*) and *wei* (protective *qi*)

Formula: Cinnamon Combination *(Gui zhi tang)*

Acu-points: Sp-2 *Dadu,* Sp-17 *Shidou,* Du-16 *Fengfu,* Lu-7 *Lieqie,*

Shaoyin Bing Zheng Syndrome

Symptoms: Desire to sleep in a curled recumbent position, abdominal aches, watery diarrhea, soft and weak abdomen, limbic heaviness, fatigue, and a minute and thready pulse

Treatment principle: Warm the kidneys

Formula: Vitality Combination *(Zhen wu tang)*

Acu-points: Ren-4 *Guanyuan*, Ren-6 *Qihai*, K-3 *Taizxi*, UB-23 *Shenshu*, P-7 *Daling*, Sp-9 *Yinlingquaan*, St-36 *Zusanli*

Cold Due to Yang Deficiency
(Han Yang Xu Zheng) (Shaoyin Bing Zheng)
Symptoms: Chills over the back, generalized aching, cold extremities, pain in limbs and joints, tastelessness, pale tongue with slippery coating, and deep pulse

Treatment principle: Warm meridians and reinforce *yang*, eliminate damp and alleviate pain

Formula: Aconite Combination *(Fu zi tang)*

Acu-points: Ren-3 *Zhongji*, Ren-4 *Guanyuan*, Sp-6 *Sanyinjiao*, Du-2 *Shenzhu*, Du-4 *Mingmen*, UB-23 *Shenshu*

Deficient Cold Separating Syndrome
(Han Cu Zheng)(Shaoyin Han Hue Zheng)
Symptoms: Diarrhea, bloody and purulent stool (with a mild odor), dysuria, dull pain in the abdomen (relieved by pressure and warmth), pale tender tongue with white slippery coating, and deep, slow and thready pulse

Treatment principle: Warm *yang* and consolidate collapse

Formula: Kaolin and Oryza Combination *(Tao hua tang)*

Acu-points: Ren-4 *Guanyuan*, Ren-6 *Qihai*, St-25 *Tianshu*, UB-17 *Geshu*, UB-20 *Pishu*, Sp-6 *Sanyinjiao*

Edema Due to Yang Deficiency
(Yin Shui Zheng) (Yin Edema)
Symptoms: Lassitude, heaviness of extremities, edema, desire to sleep, dizziness, epigastric throbbing, abdominal pain, dysuria, diarrhea, and white slippery coating on tongue, and weak pulse

Treatment principle: Warm *yang* and remove water

Formula: Vitality Combination *(Zhen wu tang)*

Acu-points: Ren-3 *Zhongji*, Ren-6 *Qihai*, Ren-12 *Zhongwan*, Sp-9 *Yinlingquan*, UB-23 *Shenshu*

Excessive Yin Repelling Yang Syndrome
(Yin Sheng Ge Yang Zheng)
Symptoms: Feverish body with flushed face, aversion to cold, curled recumbent position (when resting), cold extremities, diarrhea with undigested food, irritation of the heart, retching, deep minute pulse, or minute thready pulse (that disappears with pressure)

Treatment principle: Dispel cold, recover *yang*, and promote circulation in both the interior and exterior

Formula: White penetrating decoction *(Bai tong tang)*

Acu-points: Ren-4 *Guanyuan*, Ren-8 *Shenque*, Du-20 *Baihui*, St-36 *Zusanli*

Heat Symptoms due to Yin Deficiency

(Shaoyin Re Hua Zheng)
Symptoms: Insomnia due to irritation of the heart, dryness of the mouth, dry throat, feverish sensation in palms and soles, red tongue with little coating, and deep thready pulse

Treatment principle: Nourish *Yin*, reduce heat

Formula: Coptis and Gelatin Combination *(Huang lian e jiao tang)*

Acu-points: K-1 *Yongquan*, K-6 *Zhaohai*, H-9 *Shaochong*, SI-3 *Houxi*, P-4 *Ximan*

Retention of Cold-Fluid in the Stomach Syndrome
(Han Yin Ting Wei Zheng)
Symptoms: vomiting of clear fluid, splashing sounds in the stomach, cold extremities, loose stool, clear urine; thin-white, moist and slippery coating on tongue, and wiry, thready and slow pulse

Treatment principle: Warm the stomach, pacify counter flow and stop vomiting

Formula: Evodia Combination *(Wu zhu yu tang)*

Acu-points: Ren-12 *Zhongwan*, St-36 *Zusanli*, UB-20 *Pishu*, Per-6 *Neiguan*

Shaoyin Cold Transforming Syndrome
(Shaoyin Han Hua Zheng)
Symptoms: Desire to sleep in curled recumbent position, aversion to cold, diarrhea with undigested food, cold extremities, possible *yang* depletion, and deep minute and thready pulse

Treatment principle: Warm the middle *jiao* and remove cold and restore *yang*

Formula: Aconite, Ginger, and Licorice Combination *(Si ni tang)*

Acu-points: Ren-4 *Guanyuan*, Ren-6 *Qihai*, K-3 *Taixi*, UB-23 *Shenshu*, P-7 *Daling*

Shaoyin Heat Transforming Syndrome
(Shaoyin Re Hua Zheng)
Symptoms: Insomnia due to irritation of the heart, dryness in mouth and throat, red tongue, and deep thready pulse

Treatment principle: Nourish *yin* and clear heat

Formula: Coptis and Gelatin Combination *(Huang lian e jiao tang)* or Kaolin and Oryza Combination *(Tao hua tang)*

Acu-points: H-7 *Shenmen,* H-9 *Shaochong,* K-1 *Yongquan,* K-6 *Zhaohai,* P-4 *Ximan,* UB-15 *Xinshu*

Shaoyin with Exterior Syndrome
(Shaoyin Yu Biao Zheng) (Shaoyin Yu Taiyang Bing Zheng)
Symptoms: Fever, headache, aversion to cold, no sweating, cold extremities, white tongue coating, and deep pulse

Treatment principle: Remove cold and warm meridians, relieve exterior syndrome

Formula: Ma-huang and Asarum Combination *(Ma huang fu zi xi xin tang)*

Acu-points: SI-4 *Wangu,* Ht-5 *Tongli,* K-3 *Zhaohai,* UB-58 *Feiyang*

Shaoyin with Yangming Syndrome
(Shaoyin Yu Yangming Bing Zheng)
Symptoms: Pain in the abdomen with hard fullness, dryness in mouth and throat, constipation or watery diarrhea, red tongue, forceful, thread and rapid pulse

Treatment principle: Remove heat and restore yin

Formula: Major Rhubarb Combination *(Da cheng* qi *tang)*

Acu-points: SJ-6 *Zhigou,* St-25 *Tianshu,* St-37 *Shang juxu,* Lu-7 *Lueque,* K-6 *Zhaohai*

Water and Heat Intermingle due to Yin Deficiency
(Re Yin Xu Zheng)
Symptoms: Diarrhea, dysuria, vomiting, cough, thirst, insomnia due to irritation of the heart, red tongue with little coating, and deep rapid pulse

Treatment principle: Nourish *yin* and resolve water

Formula: Polyporus Combination *(Zhu ling tang)*

Acu-points: Sp-9 *Yinlingquan*, SI-4 *Wangu*, H-5 *Tongli*, K-3 *Taixi*, UB-20 *Pishu*

Yang Deficiency and Yin Excess
(Yang Xu Yin Shi Zheng)
Symptoms: Lassitude, desire to sleep in a curled recumbent position, cold extremities, diarrhea, vomiting with undigested food, aversion to cold, sweating, abdominal pain, pale tongue with white slippery coating, and a deep thready pulse

Treatment principle: Warm and restore *yang*

Formula: Aconite, Ginger, and Licorice Combination *Si ni tang* or Aconite, Ginseng, and Ginger Combination *(Fu zi li zhong wan)*

Acu-points: Ren-4 *Guanyuan*, Ren-6 *Qihai*, Per-6 *Neiguan*, Du-4 *Mingmen*, Du-14 *Dazhui*, UB-23 *Shenshu*

Yin Excess Dispersing Yang
(Yin Shi Kai Yang Zheng)(Shaoyin Yu Jueyin Jian Bing Zheng)
Symptoms: Diarrhea with undigested food, cold extremities, thirst (but no desire to drink), fever with no aversion to cold, flushed face, retching, sore throat, and minute pulse

Treatment principle: Restore the *yang*

Formula: Licorice, Aconite, and Ginger Pulse Combination *(Tong mai si ni tang)*

Acu-points: Ren-4 *Guanyuan*, Ren-6 *Qihai*, St-36 *Zusanli*, UB-20 *Pishu*, K-3 *Taixi*, H-7 *Shenmen*

Jueyin Bing Zheng Syndrome

Symptoms: Heat above and cold below, wasting thirst, anxiety and irritability, burning stabbing pain in epigastrium, hunger (but no appetite), chilling due to ascarasis, cold limbs, pale tongue with white coating, and weak pulse

Treatment principle: Clear the upper heat and warm the lower cold, dispel ascarasis

Formula: Mume Formula *(Wu Mei Wan)*

Acu-points: Liv-3 *Taizhong*, P-6 *Neiguan*, P-7 *Daling*, Ren-14 *Juque*, St-36 *Zusanli*

Ascaris Vomiting
(Chong Tu Zheng) (Jueyin Bing Zheng)
Symptoms: Cold extremities, wasting thirst, *qi* surging up into the heart, vomiting of roundworms on food intake, and improper use of purgation that causes continuous diarrhea

Treatment principle: Regulate cold and heat, harmonize stomach, and expel roundworms

Formula: Mume Formula *(Wu Mei Wan)*

Acu-points: Sp-4 *Gongsun*, P-6 *Neiguan*, Ren-12 *Zhongwan*, Liv-14 *Qimen*

Cold Separating Syndrome
(Jueyin Han Zheng)
Symptoms: Lasting diarrhea, abdominal pain (relieved by warmth), cold feet, frequent vomiting, vomiting upon intake of food, improper use of emetic or purgation that aggravate diarrhea and vomiting, pale tongue with thin-yellow coating, and deficient rapid pulse

Treatment principle: Clear upper heat and warm lower cold with pungent and bitter herbs

Formula: Ginger, Pinellia, and Ginseng Formula *(Gan Jian Huang Qin Huang Lian Ren Shen Tang)* also known as *Gan Jiang Ren Shen Ban Xia Wan*

Acu-points: Liv-3 *Taichong*, Sp-4 *Gongsun*, P-6 *Neiguan*, LI-4 *Hegu*, St-36 *Zusanli*, K-10 *Yingu*

Jueyin Cold Syndrome
(Jueyin Han Zheng)
Symptoms: Cold extremities, aversion to cold, no fever, spontaneous perspiration, watery diarrhea, pale tongue, and minute weak or slow pulse.

Treatment principle: Restore *yang*

Formula: Aconite, Ginger, and Licorice Combination *(Si ni tang)*

Acu-points: Ren-4 *Guanyuan*, Ren-6 *Qihai*, Du-4 *Mingmen*, Du-14 *Dazhui*, St-36 *Zusanli*

Jueyin Heat Syndrome
(Jueyin Re Zheng)
Symptoms: High fever, thirst, cold extremities, abdominal distention and fullness, irritability, fainting, yellowish or reddish urine, yellow coating on tongue, and rapid pulse

Treatment principle: Clear heat and resuscitation

Formula: Bupleurum and Chih-shih Formula *(Si ni san)*

Acu-points: LI-4 *Hegu*, LI-11 *Quchi*, St-44 *Neiting*, St-45 *Lidui*

Nausea and Retching Syndrome
(E Xin Gan Ou Zheng)
Symptoms: Vomiting, nausea and retching, sub cardiac distention and cold limbs, diarrhea, spitting saliva, headache, and sinking thin and slow pulse

Treatment principle: Warm the stomach, dispel cold, pacify counter flow and stop vomiting.

Formula: Evodia Combination *(Wu zhu yu tang)*

Acu-points: Liv-1 *Dadun*, P-6 *Neiguan*, Du-20 *Baihui*. Ren-12 *Zhongwan*, St-36 *Zhusanli*

Superior Heat and Inferior Cold
(Shang Re Xia Han Zheng) (Jueyin Bing Zheng)
Symptoms: Heat lodged in upper region with cold in lower region of the body, and cold limbs, cold limbs, pale tongue with white coating, and weak pulse

Treatment principle: Clear the upper heat and warm the lower cold

Formula: Mume Formula or Mume Pill *(Wu Mei Wan)*

Acu-points: K-1 (Yongquan), Du-20 (Baihui)

Jueyin Jian Bing Syndrome

Superior Heat, Inferior Cold with Yin Deficiency
(Shang Re Xia Han Yin Xu Zheng) (Jueyin Yu Taiyang Jian Bing)
Symptoms: Cold extremities, continuous diarrhea, swollen and painful throat, sputum with bloody pus, and deep slow pulse in the *cun* (middle) position and a non-existent pulse in the *chi* (lower) position

Treatment principle: Disperse stagnant *yang*, clear excess heat, tonify spleen, and warm inferior cold

Formula: Ma-huang and Cimicifuga Combination *(Ma huang sheng ma tang)* also known as *Shi shen tang*

Acu-points: K-1 *yongquan*, Liv-1 *Dadun*, P-6 *Neiguan*, Lu-9 *Taiyuan*

Chapter Nine

Shang Han Lun Basic Formulas (Indications and Conformations)

Overview

The main emphasis in this section is on the primary formulas from the Classic *Shang Han Lun* (Treaties on Fever and Chills) and the *Jen Kuei Yao Lue* (Prescriptions from the Golden Chamber).

- Conformations for formulas and a comparison to other formulas for each "stage"
- Twenty eight primary formulas
- Formulas listed by their English common name
- Major indications
- Precautions and contraindications

Taiyang Stage Formulas

Cinnamon Combination

Gui zhi tang is used to treat severe chills, fever, and headache.

The *Shang Han Lun* states, *"Cinnamon Combination Gui zhi tang should be given [to patients with] taiyang disease who have headaches, fever, perspiration and mild chills [anemophobia]." "When the outside confirmation of taiyang disease is not relieved by the sweating method [as evidenced by] a floating and weak pulse, Gui zhi tang (Cinnamon Combination) may be given."* This formula is more appropriate for a weaker type constitution than Pueraria Combination *(Ge gen tang)* because it is not as harsh. Patients suffering from malnutrition can be treated with Cinnamon Combination *(Gui zhi tang)* as it is indicated for a weak conformation during a *taiyang* disease in which a floating and weak pulse is felt.

Major indications: Fever, severe chills, headache, spontaneous sweats that are due to patient being weak, flushing up, convulsions, pain under the heart, floating and weak pulse, and a normal light-red tongue

Ma-huang Combination

Ma huang tang is used for treating common colds, headache, fever, general pain, and asthma. The *Shang Han Lun*, states: *"taiyang disease with [the symptoms] of headache, fever, generalized discomfort, low back pain, aging of the joints, mild chills [anemophobia], and gasping, but no perspiration, is treated with Ma huang Combination. The shang han [condition] associated with a floating and tense pulse, no perspiration, and a nosebleed should be treated primarily with Ma huang Combination Ma huang tang."*

Major indications: Stiff neck and shoulders, body ache (somatic pain), headaches, aversion to cold, no sweating, asthma, floating-tight pulse, light-red tongue, and an abdomen that is normal or soft with little resistance

Minor Bupleurum Combination

Xiao chai hu tang is used for treating those of an average constitution with chest distention, hardness beneath the heart, pain beneath the ribs (hypochondria region) when pressure is applied, resistance and pressure pain beneath the liver, loss of appetite, stress, vomiting, bitter taste in the mouth, dry throat, vertigo, and recurrent fever and chills. This is a popular formula recorded in several places in the *Shang Han Lun*. For example, *"If the shang han [condition] persists for five to six days with alternating chills and fever, distress and fullness in the chest and ribs, silence with loss of appetite disturbances in the heart with a tendency to vomit or disturbances in the chest without vomiting, thirst, abdominal aching, obstruction and stiffness beneath the ribs, or palpitations beneath the heart, dysuria, adypsia, mild generalized fever, or cough, Minor Bupleurum Combination Xiao chai hu tang is indicated."*

The *Shang Han Lun* further states, *"[Patients with a] shang han condition with an obstructed, rough pulse on superficial palpation and a tense pulse on deep touch will have an acute abdominal ache and should first take Minor Cinnamon and Paeonia Combination Xiao jian zhong tang. If recovery is not complete, Minor Bupleurum Combination Xiao chai hu tang should be taken."*

The *Jen Kuei Yao Lue* states, *"Xiao chai hu tang (Minor Bupleurum Combination) treats various jaundice conditions with vomiting and abdominal aging."*

Major indications: Common cold or febrile diseases, bronchitis, gastric weakness, hepatitis, deafness, diarrhea or constipation, lymphadenitis, anorexia, tight-thin or tight-rapid pulse, white coat on tongue, and painful-obstruction and hardening beneath the heart

Pueraria Combination

Ge gen tang is suitable for treating greater febrile or afebrile common cold with severe chills, stiffness in the neck and back, diarrhea, and severe muscle spasms. According to the *Shang Han Lun*, *"taiyang disease in which there is a sensation of stiffness and heaviness in the neck and back, mild chills [anemophobia] but no perspiration, should be given Pueraria Combination Ge gen tang is given to patients experiencing diarrhea as a complication of greater and yangming diseases."*

Shoulder stiffness with tension and stiffness down to mid-shoulder blades is a major conformation for Pueraria Combination *(Ge gen tang)*. Pain that is mainly above the shoulders into the occiput region of the neck is treated more with bupleurum *(chai hu)* related formulas. Pain more on the left side of the neck and shoulder is treated with Evodia and Pinellia Combination *(Yan nian ban xia tang)*. When shoulder pain is a result of constipation, then use Siler and Platycondon Combination *(Fang feng tong sheng san)*.

For shoulder pain due to fullness of the abdomen, formulas such as Pinellia Combination *(Ban xia xie xin tang)*, Pinellia and Licorice Combination *(Gan cao xie xin tang)* or Pinellia and Ginger Combination *(Sheng jiang xie xin tang)* may be effective. For more serious shoulder stiffness, increase the amount of pueraria *(ge gen)*. *yin* type disorders, with spontaneous sweating and stiffness and spasms in the neck and back should be treated with Cinnamon and Pueraria Combination *(Gui zhi jia ge gen tang)*. Pueraria, Coptis and Scute Combination *(Ge gen huang lian huang qin tang)* is useful for shoulder stiffness due to diarrhea. Aging in the shoulders and arms due to occluded blood and constipation is relieved by Persica and Rhubarb Combination *(Tao he cheng qi tang)*. When shoulder pain is due to gynecological disorders with stagnation of blood, use Cinnamon and Hoelen Combination *(Gui zhi fu ling wan)*.

Major indications: Painful joints, stiff painful shoulders (mainly between shoulder blades), floating-strong and fast pulse, normal tongue with a little dry-white coat or no coat, and mild tension in the lower abdomen

Yangming Stage Formulas

Coptis and Rhubarb Combination

San huang xie xin tang treats excess heat in the stomach and constipation. The *Jen Kuei Yao Lue* states, *"Coptis and Rhubarb Combination San huang xie xin tang treats a patient with deficiency of heart qi, hematemesis and nosebleeds."* This formula facilitates bile secretion and bowel evacuation.

Major indications: Habitual constipation, full sensation in chest and stomach region, palpitation, bleed easily; (i.e., nosebleed and hemorrhoidal bleeding), blood congested in the head, red face, craving to drink wine, flushing up, tinnitus, insomnia, dizziness, thirst, cold legs, big-forceful or floating-big pulse, dry tongue with yellow coat, a sensation of fullness and hardness with heat in stomach

Major Rhubarb Combination

Da cheng qi tang is used for treating patients with a strong abdomen, abdominal distention, a sensation of heaviness in the body, ephidrosis, a sinking-strong pulse, constipation, moist fever, and a dry tongue and mouth. Those with a fast-weak pulse and ascites should not take this formula.

The *Shang Han Lun* states, *"Shang han [conditions] that have not been relieved by the vomiting and purgation methods may exhibit an absence of bowel movements for five or six days, occasionally up to ten days, along with tide [fluctuating] fever at dusk without severe chills but with hallucinations. In severe cases the patient may fail to recognize others, be easily frightened, and have purposeless movements, restlessness, slight gasping respiration, fixed staring, and delirium. This indicates the need for Major Rhubarb Combination Da cheng qi tang."*

The *Shang Han Lun* further states, *"A combination of yangming and shaoyang diseases with diarrhea, smooth and rapid pulse, and undigested food remaining in the stomach can be purged as an alternate treatment with Major Rhubarb Combination Da cheng qi tang."*

The *Jen Kuei Yao Lue* states, *"A strong convulsive disease in a patient manifesting thoracic fullness, lockjaw, tetany, spasms of the feet, and involuntary gnashing of teeth may be treated with Major Rhubarb Combination Da cheng qi tang. The Jen Kuei Yao Lue further states, "Diarrhea with a slow and slippery pulse signifies a firm condition of the stomach. If the diarrhea shows no sign of ceasing, the person should be purged immediately with Major Rhubarb Combination Da cheng qi tang as the preferred formula."*

Major indications: Hard and full abdomen, heavy sensation throughout the body, high fever with constipation, delirium, sweating without chills, big and strong pulse, dry tongue with yellow coat, strong and full abdomen

> NOTE: Major Rhubarb Combination *(Da cheng qi tang)* is closely related to Major Bupleurum Combination *(Da chai hu tang)* and Siler and Platycondon Combination *(Fang feng tong sheng san)*.

Minor Rhubarb Combination

Xiao cheng qi tang is Major Rhubarb Combination *(Da cheng qi tang)* minus mirabilitum *(mang xiao)*. Major Rhubarb Combination *(Da cheng qi tang)* affects all three warmers. Minor Rhubarb Combination *(Xiao cheng qi tang)* affects mainly the middle warmer and is not as strong as Major Rhubarb Combination *(Da cheng qi tang)*.

The *Shang Han Lun* states, *"Minor Rhubarb Combination Xaio cheng qi tang may be given for cases of yangming disease with tide [fluctuating] fever and semi-solid stools. If no bowel movement results after six or seven days, the stools have probably become hard. Under these circumstances a small amount of Minor Rhubarb Combination Xiao cheng qi tang may be administered. Once the disease has affected the abdomen, gas may be passed, a sign of a hard stool. Now the patient may be treated with the purgation method. Purgation is not recommended if no gas has been passed because the stools are hard but will become soft due to treatment with Minor Rhubarb Combination Xiao cheng qi tang. If the purgation method is utilized, stomach congestion and loss of appetite will result. Furthermore, if the patient is thirsty and drinks water, hiccoughs will occur. When fever is present, the patient often has firm and scanty stools and should be harmonized with Minor Rhubarb Combination Xiao cheng qi tang. The purgation method is never advised in the absence of flatus."*

The *Jen Kuei Yao Lue* states, *"Minor Rhubarb Combination Xiao cheng qi tang treats a patient with delirium following diarrhea. This signifies the presence of dry stool.*

"Jen Kuei Yao Lue further states, *"Minor Rhubarb Combination Xiao cheng qi tang treats constipation, retching and frequent delirium."* This formula also is useful for improving kidney function.

Major indications: Generalized edema, dysuria, food stagnation (food poisoning), obesity, acute febrile diseases, sinking firm pulse, thin-yellow coat on tongue, and fullness in the abdomen

Shaoyang Stage Formulas

Atractylodes Combination
Yue bi jia shu tang is used for treating dysuria, skin problems, hydrosis, and weakness in the waist and feet. The *Jen Kuei Yao Lue* states, *"Yue bi jia shu tang (Atractylodes Combination) treats muscle exhaustion which in the presence of fever exhibits loss of body fluids, enlarged pores and muscular looseness, and profuse sweating. It also alleviates severe wind and weakness of the lower warmer and feet."*

Major indications: Edema, dermatic nephritis, nephritis, rheumatic degenerative arthritis, acute conjunctivitis, submerged pulse, normal tongue

Atractylodes and Hoelen Combination
Ling gui shu gan tang is used for treating palpitations, hyperpnoea, distention in the chest near the heart, and flushing up due to water toxins. The *Jen Kuei Yao Lue* states, *"Atractylodes and Hoelen Combination Ling gui shu gan tang relieves water stagnancy beneath the heart which manifest thoracocostal distention and dizziness."*

The *Jen Kuei Yao Lue* also states, *"Shortness of breath with mild water stagnancy has to be eliminated through urination. It requires Atractylodes and Hoelen Combination Ling gui shu gan san or Rehmania Eight Combination Ba wei ti huang tang."*

Major indications: Stomach trouble with flushing up, water in the stomach, palpitation, nervous disorders, bleeding in the eyes, tinnitus, cardiac hypo function, submerged-tense pulse, pale and swollen tongue, abdominal laxity

> **Note**: Atractylodes and Hoelen Combination *(Ling gui shu gan san)* with Tang Kuei Four Combination *(Si wu tang)* makes Tang Kuei and Atractylodes Combination *(Lien zhu yin)* and is used to treat blood *(xue)* and water *(Jinye)* disorders together. Patients with gastrointestinal weakness should not take this formula.

Bupleurum and Cinnamon Combination

Chai hu gui zhi tang is useful for those with a somewhat delicate constitution who have a tendency towards fatigue, gastrointestinal weakness, headache, heaviness in the head, neuralgia, fever, moderately severe chills, distention beneath the heart, and tenderness around the pubic bone. The *Shang Han Lun* states, *"Shang han [conditions] lasting six or seven days with fever, mild [inside] chills, persisting aging in the limbs [surface conformation], mild vomiting and distention beneath the heart require Bupleurum and Cinnamon Combination Chai hu gui zhi tang. These symptoms signify that an outside conformation still exists in the temporal areas."*

The *Jen Kuei Yao Lue* states, *"Bupleurum and Cinnamon Combination Chai hu gui zhi tang treats acute pain of the heart and the abdomen."* Bupleurum and Cinnamon Combination *(Chai hu gui zhi tang)* is a mixture of 50% Minor Bupleurum Combination *(Xiao chai hu tang)* and 50% Cinnamon Combination *(Gui zhi tang)*.

Major indications: Chest distress, abdominal distention, spontaneous sweating, epigastric knot, floating-weak and cordal pulse, or floating moderate pulse, dry-white tongue coating, tense abdominal muscles

> Note: In Japan, Bupleurum and Cinnamon Combination *(Chai hu gui zhi tang)* is commonly used for epilepsy.

Bupleurum, Cinnamon and Ginger Combination

Chai hu gui zhi gan kan jiang tang is used for treating people with a delicate constitution. The *Shang Han Lun* states, *"Shang han [conditions] lasting five to six days that have been treated first with the sweating method and then the purgation method but exhibit [continued] fullness and congestion in the chest, dysuria, thirst without vomiting, perspiration in the head area, alternating chills and fever, and anxiety should be given Bupleurum, Cinnamon and Ginger Combination Chai hu gui zhi gan jiang tang."*

The *Jen Kuei Yao Lue* states, *"Bupleurum, Cinnamon and Ginger Combination Chai hu gui zhi gan jiang tang treats malaria with chills and a mild fever or with chills and no fever [one dose of this drug produces a divine effect]."*

This formula is similar to Bupleurum and Cinnamon Combination *(Chai hu gui zhi tang)*. However, it is used for weaker patients; e.g., people who catch a cold easily or get fatigued easily.

Major indications: Epigastric fullness and hardness, palpitation above umbilicus, thirst with dry lips and mouth, dysuria, sweating forehead, flushing up, neurosis, weak-floating or floating-small pulse, wet tongue with no coating; epigastric region full and soft with a feeling of distension and sometimes succussion sounds

Bupleurum and Dragon Bone Combination

Chai hu jia long gu mu li tang -- Doctor *Zhang Zhong Jing* of the Han Dynasty commented on this formula as being a sedative which was used in harmonizing the "inside" and "outside" and sedating the mind. This formula is used for treating chest and sub cardiac distention, insomnia, irritability, melancholia, fearfulness, and tendency towards mania, and convulsion.

The *Shang Han Lun* states, *"[The patient still suffering from] a shang han [condition] for eight or nine days after treatment with the purgation method [with a feeling of] fullness in the chest, anxiety and nervousness, dysuria, delirium, heaviness of body, and difficulty in turning should be treated mainly with Bupleurum and Dragon Bone Combination Chai hu jia long gu mu li tang."*

Major indications: Anxiety, chest distress, palpitations near or above the umbilicus, hyper function of the heart, constipation, decreased urination, flushing up, neurosis, neurotic insomnia, sinking-tight pulse, dry tongue with slight white coat, strong palpitation above umbilicus

> Note: The original formula contained lead oxide PBO, which is very toxic. Three hundred years later the PBO has been discontinued. Bupleurum and Dragon Bone Combination *(Chai hu jia long gu mu li tang)* and Bupleurum Combination *(Yi gan san)* are both used for the same basic symptoms; however, Bupleurum and Dragon Bone Combination *(Chai hu jia long gu mu li tang)* is used for stronger conformations. Bupleurum Combination *(Yi gan san)* is used for conformation that is between strong and weak.

Capillaris Combination

Yin chen hao tang is a major formula for treating jaundice, constipation, and dark colored urine. The *Shang Han Lun* states, *"Shang han [conditions] that have lasted for seven to eight days with a yellow-orange coloration of the skin (jaundice), dysuria, a tendency towards constipation, and mild congestion in the abdomen should be treated mainly with yin chen hao tang (Capillaris Combination). For cases without constipation yin chen wu ling tang (Capillaris and Hoelen Combination) is recommended."*

The *Jen Kuei Yao Lue* states, *"Chills and fever which cause anorexia, dizziness after eating, and discomfort in the heart and chest portend gu tan (cereal jaundice). The afflicted primarily needs yin chen hao tang (Capillaris Combination)."*

Major indications: Jaundice with chest distention, acute hepatitis, a sensation of vomiting, oliguria even though the patient has drunk water, food poisoning, uticaria, sunken-firm pulse, yellow coat on tongue, fullness in abdomen

Hoelen Five Herb Combination

Wu ling san is used for stagnant water in the stomach due to a metabolic disorder, thirst, vomiting, and dysuria, flushing up, palpitations, vertigo, anxiety, headache, abdominal pain, diarrhea, edema, and fever. The *Shang Han Lun* states, *"Hoelen Five Herb Combination Wu ling san is recommended [for patients] with a floating and rapid pulse, distress, and thirst after perspiring."*

The Jen Kuei Yao Lue states, "A thin individual who has palpitation beneath the navel, slobbering, and dizziness has a water problem and needs Hoelen Five Herb Combination Wu ling san."

Major indications: Thirst, vomiting, dysuria, watery diarrhea, stagnant water in the stomach due to metabolic disorder, floating-slippery and fast pulse, dry tongue with a yellow coat, and painful abdomen

Major Bupleurum Combination

Da chai hu tang is used for those having obese or strong constitution with good skin, strong and sunken pulse, pains in the chest, habitual constipation, diarrhea, vomiting, asthma, mental instability, and a tendency towards irritability. This formula is used for more severe symptoms than those treated by Minor Bupleurum Combination *(Xiao chai hu tang)*.

The Shang Hun Lun states, "Sometimes taiyang disease persists for more than ten days and moves slowly into the shaoyang stage. If it has been mistakenly treated with two or three purgations [under the assumption that the disease has shifted to the yangming stage] and four or five days later it still exhibits Chai hu tang (Bupleurum Conformation), it should now be treated with Minor Bupleurum Combination Xiao chai hu tang. In cases of severe vomiting [after taking this combination], plus unrelieved stagnancy beneath the heart and distress in the chest, treatment with Major Bupleurum Combination Da chai hu tang may result in recovery after an episode of diarrhea."

The *Jen Kuei Yao Lue* states, *"Distention and aching beneath the heart due to firm evil should be purged with Major Bupleurum Combination Da chai hu tang as the preferred drug."*

Major indications: Epigastric distress, strong type constitution with good color and strong voice, heavy head sensation, anger easily, alternating chill and fever, gallstones, asthma, hypertension, sunken-strong or sunken-slow pulse; can also be tight and big; dry tongue with white or yellow coat; abdominal tension with discomfort upon pressure

Ma huang and Apricot Seed Combination

Ma xing gan shi tang is a simple but strong formula. This formula is used for treating fever due to stagnant heat in the lungs as well as thirst, and wheezing. The *Shang Han Lun* states, *"[The patient] who gasps after perspiring should not be given additional Gui zhi tang (Cinnamon Combination). Those without a severe fever [who are subjected to] gasping after perspiring may be given Ma xing gan shi tang (Apricot Seed and Ma huang Combination)."*

Main indications: Gasping cough, whooping cough in children, children with asthma, cough with sweating and thirst, fever with no chills, floating-quick pulse, red tongue with white coat

> Note: A ratio of 50% *Ma huang* and Apricot Seed Combination *(Ma xing gan shi tang)* plus 50% Minor Blue Dragon Combination *(Xiao qing long tang)* may be used for a gasping cough with a red face, or a severe cough that causes asthma. Dosage should be administered 1-2 times a day.

> *Ma huang* (ephedra) is used mainly for disease in the *yang* stage. Some formulas that contain *ma huang*, however, may be used to treat disease that has penetrated deeper into the muscle, causing edema and thus becoming a *yin* stage disease. In the *Shang Han Lun* it is found, *"For patients contracting shaoyin disease with fever [a symptom of taiyang disease] and a sinking pulse, Ma huang, Aconite and Asarum Combination Ma huang fu zi xi xin tang is indicated. Shaoyin disease lasting for two to three days with no sign of the inside conformation should be treated with Ma huang, Aconite*

and Licorice Combination Ma huang fu zi zi gan cao tang to render mild sweating."

Minor Bupleurum Combination

Xiao chai hu tang is used for treating those of an average constitution with chest distention, hardness beneath the heart, pain beneath the ribs (hypochondria region) when pressure is applied, resistance and pressure pain beneath the liver, loss of appetite, stress, vomiting, bitter taste in the mouth, dry throat, vertigo, and recurrent fever and chills. This is a popular formula recorded in several places in the *Shang Han Lun*. For example, *"If the shang han [condition] persists for five to six days with alternating chills and fever, distress and fullness in the chest and ribs, silence with loss of appetite disturbances in the heart with a tendency to vomit or disturbances in the chest without vomiting, thirst, abdominal aging, obstruction and stiffness beneath the ribs, or palpitations beneath the heart, dysuria, adypsia, mild generalized fever, or cough, Minor Bupleurum Combination Xiao chai hu tang is indicated."*

The *Shang Han Lun* further states, *"[Patients with a] shang han condition with an obstructed, rough pulse on superficial palpation and a tense pulse on deep touch will have an acute abdominal ache and should first take Minor Cinnamon and Paeonia Combination Xiao jian zhong tang. If recovery is not complete, Minor Bupleurum Combination Xiao chai hu tang should be taken."* The *Jen Kuei Yao Lue* states, *"Xiao chai hu tang (Minor Bupleurum Combination) treats various jaundice conditions with vomiting and abdominal aging."*

Major indications: Common cold or febrile diseases, bronchitis, gastric weakness, hepatitis, deafness, diarrhea or constipation, lymphadenitis, anorexia, thigh-thin or tight-rapid pulse, white coat on tongue, and painful-obstruction and hardening beneath the heart

Pinellia Combination

Ban xia xie xin tang is a commonly used formula for treating gastrointestinal disorders, such as, sub cardiac distention, vomiting, nausea, anorexia, resistance below the heart, ascites, borborygmus, and diarrhea. The *Shang Han Lun* states, *"Here is a comparison of the herb prescriptions Bupleurum Formula Chai hu tang known as Yi gan san, Rhubarb and Kan-sui Combination Da xian xiong tang, and Pinellia Combination Ban xia xie xin tang in the treatment of shan han [conditions]. Shan han [conditions] of the bupleurum chai hu confirmation present vomiting and fever lasting five to six days even following purging by another herb. Bupleurum Combination Yi gan san initiates shivering followed by fever and perspiration, which alleviates [the problem]. If there is congestion with hardness and pain beneath the heart, Rhubarb and Kan-sai Combination Da xian xiong tang is indicated. For cases with congestion beneath the heart without pain, Pinellia Combination Ban xia xie xin tang is recommended rather than Bupleurum Formula Yi gan san."*

The *Jen Kuei Yao Lue* states, *"Pinellia Combination Ban xia xie xin tang treats vomiting combined with borborygmus and obstruction beneath the heart."* This formula is similar to Coptis Combination *(Huang lien tang).* The difference is that cinnamon is taken out and scute *(huang qin)* is added which makes the formula better for heat in the stomach and irritability in the chest.

Major indications: *Shaoyang* disorders, vomiting, dry heaves, borborygmus, heat and water accumulation in the stomach, all kinds of stomach disease, diarrhea with no fever, nausea, gastritis, no appetite, tight-sinking or tight-weak pulse, dry tongue with a slightly wet and white coat, a sensation of abdominal fullness which is painful upon pressure

Polyporus Combination

Zhu ling tang is used for treating difficult and painful urination, dysuria with thirst, and fullness and pain in the lower abdomen. The *Jen Kuei Yao Lue* states, *"When the cause of the disease is located above the diaphragm and vomiting followed by a desire to drink water occurs, it means that the patient is going to recover. A little water should be given immediately. Polyporus Combination Zhu ling tang slakes excessive thirst."*

Major indications: Lower abdominal heat, urinary tract inflammation, painful decreased urination, extreme thirst, sensation of holding urine after voiding, hematuria, kidney stones, cystitis, toxemia, neurosis (insomnia), diarrhea, edema, floating pulse, dry-red tongue, tense lower abdomen

Taiyin Stage Formulas

Cinnamon and Peony Combination

Gui zhi jia shao yao tang is used for treating a patient of a delicate constitution with abdominal pain, diarrhea, abdominal distention, and spasms in the abdomen. The *Shang Han Lun* states, *"taiyang disease that should have been treated by the sweating method but instead was treated by the purgation method with resultant continued abdominal congestion and occasional aging should be given Cinnamon and Peaonia Combination Gui zhi shao yao tang."*

> Note: Peony *(shao yao)* changes the cinnamon formula by directing the effect more to the middle *san jiao* (triple warmer) area. Normally cinnamon formulas are used for more "surface" symptoms. The addition of *shao yao* causes the formula to have a more internal effect.

Major indications: T*aiyang* stage moving towards *yin* stage, intermittent abdominal pain and fullness, hypochondriac pain (right side), headache, fever, mild shoulder stiffness, mild diarrhea, enteritis, appendicitis, peritonitis, thin-white tongue coating, floating-fast pulse

Major Zanthoxylum Combination

Da jian zhong tang is used to dispel chills and break up obstructions, hence relieving pain in the upper as well as the lower parts of the body. The *Wai Tai Mi Yao* by *Wang Tau* states, *"Major Zanthoxylum Combination Da jian zhong tang is indicated essentially for "chill hernia", a painful heart which feels as though it is being stung, abdominal pain around the umbilicus and in the abdomen, spontaneous perspiration that is so profuse the patient feels as if he is going to die."*

Major indications: Movement in the intestines that can be observed, moving pain around the umbilicus, cold limbs, abdominal pain with a cold sensation, hyper function of the intestines, diarrhea, rabbit stools, gastropisis, intestinal hernia, retained gas in the intestines, kidney or gall stones, weak pulse, thick-white coat on tongue, abdominal weakness

> Note: Minor Cinnamon and Peony Combination *(Xiao jian zhong tang)* plus Major Zanthoxylum Combination *(Da jian zhong tang)* makes a middle of the road formula.

Minor Cinnamon and Peony Combination

Xiao jian zhong tang is to be taken by those of delicate constitution with a tendency towards fatigue. The *Shang Han Lun* states, *"Shan han [conditions continuing) for two or three days with rapid heart palpitations and distress [which cannot be treated with the sweating method due to deficiency of yang] should be treated primarily with Minor Cinnamon and Paeonia Combination Xiao jian zhong tang."*

"Jen Kuei Yao Lue states, *"Weakness, fatigue and internal cramps together with cardiac palpitation, nosebleeds, abdominal aches, nocturnal emission, soreness and aging in the extremities, fever in the limbs and dry throat and mouth are primarily treated with Minor Cinnamon and Paeonia Combination Xiao jian zhong tang."* The main herb in this formula is maltose *(jiao yi)* that supplements nutrition.

Major indications: Weakness and fatigue, fear of cold, polyuria, dry mouth and tongue, palpitations, nosebleeds, diarrhea, hot palms (weak conformation), weak pulse, dry tongue, painful abdomen

Note: Peony *(shao yao)* and maltose *(jiao yi)* are two major herbs for malnutrition in children who have symptoms of bed-wetting, painful abdomen, loose muscles (weak conformation), prolapsed rectum, tuberculosis, and peritonitis

Shaoyin Stage Formulas

Ma huang, Aconite and Asarum Combination

Ma huang fu zi xi xin tang is used for treating older or debilitated patients at the onset of a disease with symptoms of cough, expectoration of water-like thin sputum, light colored urine, anemia, and lack of vigor. The *Shang Han Lun* states, *"For patients contracting shaoyin disease with fever (a symptom of taiyang disease) and a sinking pulse, Ma huang fu zi xi xin tang (Ma huang, Aconite, and Asarum Combination) is indicated."*

Major indications: Internal water stagnation, *shaoyin* disease with fever and a small-sinking pulse, shortness of breath, weak body conformation, lack of vigor, cough and asthma, neuralgia, sinking-small and weak pulse, wet tongue without coating

Minor Pinellia and Hoelen Combination

Xiao ban xia jia fu ling tang is used for treating vomiting due to stagnant water in the stomach, sub cardiac distention, nausea, vertigo, and palpitation. The *Jen Kuei Yao Lue* states, *"The conformation of sudden vomiting, distention beneath the heart, water at the diaphragm, dizziness, and palpitation should be treated essentially with Xiao ban xia jia fu ling tang (Minor Pinellia and Hoelen Combination)."*

Major indications: Pernicious vomiting, acute gastroenteritis, gastroptosis, beriberi, extreme thirst, mild chills in hands and feet, pleurisy, thin pulse, dry and cracked tongue, abdominal weakness with water stagnation in the stomach

Vitality Combination

Zhen wu tang is mainly used to treat metabolic disorders, dysuria due to stagnant water, abdominal pain, diarrhea, vertigo, palpitation, abdominal weakness, severe fatigue, cold hands and feet, and pain in the arms and legs. The Shang *Han Lun* states, *"If the patient continues to have a fever, rapid heart palpitation, vertigo, trembling, and a tendency to collapse after perspiring which has been induced by the sweating method, he still has a taiyang disease and should be treated mainly with Vitality Combination Zhen wu tang."* and *"shaoyin disease persisting from two to five days with abdominal discomfort, difficulty in urination, heaviness and aging of the limbs, diarrhea, cough, excessive urination, constipation, and vomiting should be treated with Vitality Combination Zhen wu tang."*

Major indications: *Taiyin-shaoyin* disorders, weak fever, continuous low grade fever, exhaustion, poor digestion, water stagnation in the stomach, dizziness and vertigo, palpitation, vomiting, chronic diarrhea, distended stomach (false fullness), submerged-minute or floating-weak pulse, moist tongue with white or pale black coat; painful, soft, weak, and distended abdomen

Jueyin Stage Formulas

Aconite and G. L. Combination

Si ni tang is used for treating cold hands and feet, severe chills throughout the body, pallor, diarrhea, vomiting, abdominal pain, weak pulse, facial redness, and superficial fever. The *Shang Han Lun* states, *"shaoyin disease with a feeble, small, and sinking pulse where the chill has entered the viscera should be warmed without delay and then treated with Aconite, Ginger, and Licorice Combination Si ni tang."*

The *Shang Han Lun* also states, *"Patients with severe perspiration resulting from inappropriate therapy, retention of heat within the body [a yin confirmation that has transformed from taiyang or yangming disease], abdominal spasms, aging and coldness of the limbs, diarrhea, and severe chills should be treated with Aconite and G. L. Combination Si ni tang."* . . . *"Vomiting, diarrhea, perspiration, exhaustion of vitality, fever, severe chills, spasms of the limbs, and coldness of the hands and feet should be treated with Aconite and G. L. Combination Si ni tang."*

The <u>*Jen Kuei Yao Lue*</u> states, *"Aconite, Ginger, and Licorice Combination Si ni tang relieves vomiting, a weak pulse, frequent urination, and slight generalized fever in a person with chills. The condition is difficult to cure."*

Major indications: Surface fever interior chill, spontaneous sweating, cold arms and legs, stomach cold and weak, generalized body pain, diarrhea, influenza, neurotic vomiting; weak, minute or slow pulse; normal tongue, weak and adynamic abdomen

Licorice, Aconite, and Ginger Pulse Combination

Tong mai si ni tang is used for treating Aconite and G. L. Combination *(Si ni tang)* conformation, in which vomiting, diarrhea, and cold limbs are extremely severe and the pulse is failing rapidly. The *Shang Han Lun* states, *"For patients with shaoyin disease who have diarrhea containing undigested food; inside chills and outside fever; coldness of the hands and feet; a feeble, weak, and dying-out pulse; severe chills; ruddy face; abdominal discomfort; retching; sore throat; and a nearly imperceptible pulse that does not change after a cessation of diarrhea, Tong mai si ni tang (Aconite, Ginger, and Licorice Pulse Combination) is given."*

The *Jen Kuei Yao Lue* states, *"A patient with lientery, internal chills and external fever, and perspiration and chilling needs Tong mai si ni tang (Aconite, Ginger, Licorice Combination Fortified)."*

Major indications: Influenza, typhoid fever, autointoxication, appendicitis, gastrointestinal inflammation, dyspepsia, jaundice, hyperhydrosis, floating-weak pulse, normal tongue, and painful abdomen

Mume Formula

Wu mei wan is used primarily to expel parasites, relieves pain and diarrhea. This formula is useful for intestinal colic and ulcerative colitis. The *Shang Han Lun* states, *"Shang han conditions with a feeble and pulse and coldness of limbs persisting for seven to eight days, followed by coldness of the skin, agitation, and restlessness, does not indicate the coldness of the limbs is due to intestinal worms but instead shows a marked case of organ coldness. The patient with worms appears quiet but has frequent attacks of discomfort that subside quickly (because the worm ascends up through the diaphragm). If the patient experiences nausea following food intake, recurrent anxiety, and a vomiting of worms, the coldness of the limbs is due to worm infestation, an indication of absolute yin disease, and is best treated with Wu-mei yuan (Mume Formula).*

Major indications: Abdominal pain with vomiting of ascariasis, intermittent fever and chills, anxiety and irritability, diarrhea, cold limbs, loss of appetite, a sensation of heavy pressure in the stomach, stabbing pain below the heart, accompanied by heat above the waist and cold below

Chapter Ten

Herbal Formula (Tables)

Overview

The main emphasis in this section is on ninety one tables of herbal formulas and is designed as a quick clinical reference. Formulas are listed in alphabetical order using their common name first. The numbers for the composition are in grams.

Each table contains:

- Common name
- Pinyin spelling for the formulas
- Wade-Giles spelling (in parentheses)
- Literal translation (underlined)
- Basic clinical symptoms and signs
- Traditional function
- Contraindications
- Composition

Aconite Combination

Aconite Combination *Fu zi tang* *(Fu-tzu-tang)*	Prepared Aconite Formula
Classification	*Qu han ji:* Chill Dispelling, Warm and Transform Water and Dampness
Traditional Function	Dispels cold and dampness by warming kidneys and increase spleen *yang*
Six Stage Relationship	*Shaoyin-Jueyin, qi* level
Pulse	Thready and deep
Tongue	Moist, white coat
Abdomen	Painful
Signs and Symptoms	Cold-*Bi* syndrome, anemia, edema, abdominal pain due to chills, cold-numbness in hands and feet, apoplexy, facial paralysis, palpitations below the diaphragm, perspiration, diarrhea, decreased urine, and neuralgia
Contraindication	*Yin* deficiency

Aconite Combination (Composition)

0.5-1.0	*Fu zi (hei)*	Prepared Sichuan aconite root	*Lateralis aconiti carmichaeli radix praeparata*
5.0	*Bai zhu*	White Atractylodes root	*Atractylodis macrocephalae rhizoma*
4.0	*Fu ling*	Hoelen, Tuckahoe	*Poriae cocos sclerotium*
3.0	*Ren shen*	Ginseng root	*Ginseng radix*
4.0	*Shao yao*	Peony	*Paeoniae radix*

Atractylodes Combination

Atractylodes Combination *Yue bi jia zhu tang* *(Yueh-pe-chia-chu-tang)*	Maidservant from Yue Decoction plus Atractylodes
Classification	*Li shi ji:* Moisture Dispelling, Clear Heat form the Organs
Traditional Function	Regulates and dispels water stagnation and reduces swelling due to wind-heat
Six Stage Relationship	*Taiyang-Taiyin,* water level
Pulse	Superficial and slippery or deep
Tongue	Red-dry, thin white coat
Abdomen	Firm
Signs and Symptoms	Spontaneous sweating, jaundice, extreme thirst, hard stools, decreased urine, fever and chills, painful hands and feet with edema, dermatic nephritis, and difficult breathing with weakness in the waist and feet
Contraindication	*Yang* deficiency

Atractylodes Combination (Composition)

4.0	*Bai zhu*	White Atractylodes root	*Atractylodis macrocephalae rhizoma*
6.0	*Ma huang*	Ephedra	*Epherdrae herba*
8.0	*Shi gao*	Gypsum	*Gypsum fibrosum*
3.0	*Sheng jiang*	Fresh ginger root	*Zingiberis officinalis recens rhizoma*
3.0	*Da zao*	Red date, Jujube fruit	*Ziziphi jujubae fructus*
2.0	*Gan cao*	Licorice root	*Glycyrrhizae uralensis radix*

Bamboo and Ginseng Combination

Bamboo and Ginseng Combination *Zhu ru wen dan tang* *(Chu-ju-wen-tan-tang)*	Warm the Gall Bladder Decoction with Bamboo shavings
Classification	*He jie ji:* Harmonizing
Traditional Function	Treats febrile disease with lingering fever, clears heat in heart and gall bladder, regulates *qi* and phlegm in middle-upper *jiaos*
Six Stage Relationship	*Shaoyang,* water level
Pulse	Superficial and slippery or deep
Tongue	Red with white coat
Abdomen	Weak and soft
Signs and Symptoms	Palpitations and insomnia, tendency to startle, depressed feeling and irritability in the chest, lingering fever with copious phlegm, facial flushing
Contraindication	Excess heat conditions

Bamboo and Ginseng Combination (Composition)

3.0	*Ban xia (fa)*	Pinellia rhizome	*Pinelliae ternatae rhizoma*
1.0	*Zhi shi*	Immature bitter orange fruit	*Citri seu ponciri immaturus fructus*
1.0	*Gan jiang*	Dried ginger rhizome	*Zingiberis officinalis rhizoma*
1.0	*Chen pi*	Tangerine peel	*Citri reticulatae pericarpium*
3.0	*Jie geng (ku)*	Balloon flower root, Platycodon	*Platycodi grandiflori radix*
3.0	*Zhu ru*	Bamboo shavings	*Bambusae in taenilis caulis*
2.0	*Huang lian*	Coptis rhizome	*Coptidis rhizoma*
5.0	*Chai hu*	Bupleurum root	*Bupleuri radix*
2.0	*Ren shen*	Ginseng root	*Ginseng radix*
3.0	*Fu ling*	Hoelen, Tuckahoe	*Poriae cocos sclerotium*
2.0	*Xiang fu zi*	Scophularia root, Figwort root	*Scrophulariae ningpoensis radix*
1.0	*Gan cao*	Licorice root	*Glycyrrhizae uralensis radix*

Bamboo and Hoelen Combination

Bamboo and Hoelen Combination *Wen dan tang* *(Wen-tan-tang)*	Warm the Gall Bladder Decoction
Classification	*He jie ji:* Harmonizing
Traditional Function	Relieves exterior fever and internal water stagnation, harmonizes the stomach, relieves vomiting and dispels stomach-water stagnation
Six Stage Relationship	*Shaoyang,* water level
Pulse	Weak, floating-slippery and rapid
Tongue	Thick-white or greasy coat, may be swollen
Abdomen	Soft with sucussion sounds, tenderness below the diaphragm, and palpations below umbilicus
Signs and Symptoms	Gastric distress, palpitations and insomnia, gasping, vomiting, spontaneous sweating, cardiac edema, night sweats, weakness and pain after illness, toxemia during pregnancy, diabetes, and sea sickness
Contraindication	Excess cold conditions

Bamboo and Hoelen Combination (Composition)

6.0	*Ban xia (fa)*	Pinellia rhizome	*Pinelliae ternatae rhizoma*
6.0	*Fu ling*	Hoelen, Tuckahoe	*Poriae cocos sclerotium*
2.5	*Chen pi*	Tangerine peel	*Citri reticulatae pericarpium*
3.0	*Sheng jiang*	Fresh ginger root	*Zingiberis officinalis recens rhizoma*
2.0	*Zhu ru*	Bamboo shavings	*Bambusae in taenilis caulis*
1.5	*Zhi shi*	Immature bitter orange fruit	*Citri seu ponciri immaturus fructus*
1.0	*Huang lian*	Coptis rhizome	*Coptidis rhizoma*
3.0	*Suan zao ren*	Ziziphus seed, Sour jujube	*Zizyphi spinosae semen*

Bamboo Leaves and Gypsum Combination

Bamboo Leaves and Gypsum Combination *Zhu ye shi gao tang* *(Chu-yeh-shih-kao-tang)*	Lophatherus and Gypsum Decoction
Classification	*Qing shu ji*, Summer-Heat Dispelling
Traditional Function	Clears heat, relieves *qi* stagnation and irritability in the chest, increase *qi* and *yin*
Six Stage Relationship	*Yangming, qi* level
Pulse	Weak and rapid
Tongue	Red with white coat
Abdomen	Soft with tenderness below the diaphragm
Signs and Symptoms	Delicate constitution, loss of appetite, extreme thirst, nausea or vomiting, dry skin, dehydration, hard stools, dry mouth, profuse night sweats, insomnia and nightmares, gasping cough, discomfort in the chest, pneumonia, tuberculosis, and measles
Contraindication	Excess cold conditions

Bamboo Leaves and Gypsum Combination (Composition)

2.0	*Zhu ye*	Bamboo leaves	*Bambusae folium*
10.0	*Shi gao*	Gypsum	*Gypsum fibrosum*
3.0	*Ren shen*	Ginseng root	*Ginseng radix*
6.0	*Jing mi*	Rice grain	*Oryzae sativae semen*
2.0	*Gan cao*	Licorice root	*Glycyrrhizae uralensis radix*
6.0	*Mai men dong*	Ophiopogon tuber, Creeping lily-turf tuber	*Ophiopogonis japonici tuber*
4.0	*Ban xia (fa)*	Pinellia rhizome	*Pinelliae ternatae rhizoma*

Bupleurum Combination

Bupleurum Combination *Yi gan san* *(I-kan-san) also* *(Chai-hu-tang)*	Restrain the Liver Powder
Classification	*Zhen jing ji:* Sedative, Regulate and Harmonize Liver and Spleen
Traditional Function	Liver and spleen blood deficiency with liver-fire raising, disperse stagnant qi and relieve spasms
Six Stage Relationship	*Shaoyang, qi* and blood levels
Pulse	Thin-wiry and rapid
Tongue	Pale, purplish, thin-white coat
Abdomen	Weak with spasms and palpitations on left side, tenderness below the diaphragm
Signs and Symptoms	Weak constitution, general lassitude, nervousness, excitability, insomnia, epilepsy, rapid heart palpitations due to fear, loss of appetite, grinding of teeth, and numbness and spasms in limbs
Contraindication	*Yang* deficiency

Bupleurum Formula (Composition)

3.0	*Gou teng*	Gambir stem and hooks	*Uncariae cum uncis ramulus*
2.0	*Chai hu*	Bupleurum root	*Bupleuri radix*
3.0	*Dang gui*	Tang kuei root	*Angelicae sinensis radix*
3.0	*Chuan xiong*	Szechuan lovage root	*Ligustici chuanxiong radix*
4.0	*Fu ling*	Hoelen, Tuckahoe	*Poriae cocos sclerotium*
4.0	*Bai zhu*	White Atractylodes root	*Atractylodis macrocephalae rhizoma*
1.5	*Gan cao*	Licorice root	*Glycyrrhizae uralensis radix*

Bupleurum and Chih-shih Combination

Bupleurum and Chih-shih Combination *Si ni san* *(Szu-ni-san)*	Frigid Extremities Powder
Classification	*He jie ji:* Harmonizing, Regulate and Harmonize Liver and Spleen
Traditional Function	Soothes the liver, regulates and relieves qi stagnation, treats chest distention, improves circulation to hands and feet
Six Stage Relationship	*Shaoyang, qi* level
Pulse	Tight
Tongue	Lack of fur
Abdomen	Hardening below the costal region, abdominal distension and pain, spasms of rectus abdominis
Signs and Symptoms	Cold hands and feet, chest and abdominal fullness and distention, body aches, mental instability, night sweats, an irregular fever, dysuria, and feverish sensation in the heart area, palms and soles
Contraindication	*Yang* excess

Bupleurum and Chih-shih Combination (Composition)

5.0	*Chai hu*	Bupleurum root	*Bupleuri radix*
2.0	*Zhi shi*	Immature bitter orange fruit	*Citri seu ponciri immaturus fructus*
4.0	*Shao yao*	Peony	*Paeoniae radix*
1.5	*Gan cao*	Licorice root	*Glycyrrhizae uralensis radix*

Bupleurum and Cinnamon Combination

Bupleurum and Cinnamon Combination *Chai hu Gui zhi tang* *(Chai-hu-kuei-chih-tang)*	Bupleurum and Cinnamon Twig Decoction
Classification	*Biao li shuang jie ji:* Exterior and Interior Attacking, Harmonizing Lesser *Yang*-Stage Disorders
Traditional Function	Dispels external wind symptoms, regulates *ying* and *wei qi* by harmonizing exterior and interior
Six Stage Relationship	*Taiyang-shaoyang, qi* level
Pulse	Floating and weak
Tongue	Thin-white coat, red and quivering, or pale with scalloped edges
Abdomen	Mild distress and distension below the diaphragm, rectus abdominus tension, or flaccid and distended
Signs and Symptoms	Delicate constitution, fatigue, fever with mild chills, gastrointestinal weakness, acute pain below the heart, mild vomiting, heavy sensation in head, arthritic pain, jaundice, intercostal neuralgia, hepatitis, cholecystitis, and chronic appendicitis
Contraindication	*Yin* deficiency

Bupleurum and Cinnamon Combination (Composition)

5.0	*Chai hu*	Bupleurum root	*Bupleuri radix*
2.0	*Huang lian*	Coptis rhizome	*Coptidis rhizoma*
2.0	*Ren shen*	Ginseng root	*Ginseng radix*
4.0	*Ban xia (fa)*	Pinellia rhizome	*Pinelliae ternatae rhizoma*
2.5	*Gui zhi*	Cinnamon twig	*Cinnamomi cassiae ramulus*
2.5	*Shao yao*	Peony	*Paeoniae radix*
2.0	*Da zao*	Red date, Jujube fruit	*Ziziphi jujubae fructus*
1.0	*Gan jiang*	Dried ginger rhizome	*Zingiberis officinalis rhizoma*
1.5	*Gan cao*	Licorice root	*Glycyrrhizae uralensis radix*

Bupleurum, Cinnamon, and Ginger Combination

Bupleurum, Cinnamon, and Ginger Combination *Chai hu gui zhi jiang tang (Chai-hu-kuei-chih-kan-chiang-tang)*	Bupleurum, Cinnamon Twig, and Ginger Decoction
Classification	*He jie ji:* Harmonizing, Harmonizing Lesser Yang-Stage Disorders
Traditional Function	Treats those with a delicate constitution having recurrent fever and chills; harmonizes exterior cold and interior heat symptoms
Six Stage Relationship	*Shaoyang, qi* level
Pulse	Minute, thin and rapid
Tongue	Pale, thick-white coat
Abdomen	Soft and weak, palpitations above the umbilicus, tension and soreness below the diaphragm
Signs and Symptoms	Alternating chills and fever, head sweats, extreme thirst, discomfort in the chest, cardiac hyper-function, palpitations, insomnia, cold hands and feet, soft stools or diarrhea, decreased urine, chills around the waist and feet, hepatitis or cholecystitis with general deficient-yang symptoms, and bronchitis with gasping and dry cough
Contraindication	*Yang* excess

Bupleurum, Cinnamon, and Ginger Combination (Composition)

6.0	Chai hu	Bupleurum root	Bupleuri radix
3.0	Huang lian	Coptis rhizome	Coptidis rhizoma
3.0	Gua lou gen	Tricosanthes root	Trichosanthis radix
3.0	Gui zhi	Cinnamon twig	Cinnamomi cassiae ramulus
3.0	Mu li	Oyster shell	Ostreae concha
2.0	Gan jiang	Dried ginger rhizome	Zingiberis officinalis rhizoma
2.0	Gan cao	Licorice root	Glycyrrhizae uralensis radix

Bupleurum and Dragon Bone Combination

Bupleurum and Dragon Bone Combination *Chai hu jia long gu mu li tang (Chai-hu-chia-lung-ku-mu-li-tang)*	Bupleurum plus Dragon Bone and Oyster Shell Decoction
Classification	*Zhen jing ji:* Sedative, Sedate and Calm the Spirit
Traditional Function	Pacifies *shen* (spirit) and calms the mind, harmonizes external and internal symptoms
Six Stage Relationship	*Shaoyang, qi* level
Pulse	Tight and rapid
Tongue	Red with white coat or yellow coat
Abdomen	Resistance and distention below the diaphragm, palpitations above the umbilicus
Signs and Symptoms	Emotional instability, nervousness, tearfulness, neurotic palpitations, dysuria, constipation, sensation of heaviness in the whole body causing motor dysfunction, chest and sub cardiac distention, irritability and easily frightened, hypertension, angina pectoris, menopausal disorders, constipation, and dysuria
Contraindication	Use with caution during pregnancy

Bupleurum and Dragon Bone Combination (Composition)

5.0	*Chai hu*	Bupleurum root	*Bupleuri radix*
2.5	*Huang qin*	Skullcap root, Scute	*Scutellariae baicalensis radix*
2.5	*Long gu*	Dragon bone	*Os draconis*
2.5	*Mu li*	Oyster shell	*Ostreae concha*
3.0	*Gui zhi*	Cinnamon twig	*Cinnamomi cassiae ramulus*
3.0	*Fu ling*	Hoelen, Tuckahoe	*Poriae cocos sclerotium*
4.0	*Ban xia (fa)*	Pinellia rhizome	*Pinelliae ternatae rhizoma*
2.5	*Sheng jiang*	Fresh ginger root	*Zingiberis officinalis recens rhizoma*
1.0	*Da huang*	Rhubarb root	*Rhei radix et rhizoma*
2.5	*Ren shen*	Ginseng root	*Ginseng radix*
2.5	*Da zao*	Red date, Jujube fruit	*Ziziphi jujubae fructus*

Bupleurum and Peony Combination

Bupleurum and Peony Combination *Jia wei xiao yao san (Chia-wei-hsiao-yao-san)*	Augmented Rambling Powder
Classification	*He jie ji:* Harmonizing, Regulate and Harmonize Liver and Spleen
Traditional Function	Gynecological disorders, irregular menstruation, mental instability, cirrhosis and abdominal tenseness, thirst with persistent bitter taste in mouth; increase liver and spleen by moving *qi* and blood stagnation, and purges liver fire
Six Stage Relationship	*Shaoyang,* blood level
Pulse	Wiry and rapid
Tongue	Red sides, light purple, thin-white coat
Abdomen	Thoraco-costal distress and abdominal pain and distention
Signs and Symptoms	Body aches, night sweats, feverish sensation in cardiac area, palms and soles, dark colored urine, sensation of incomplete urination, headache, irritability, insomnia, weakness in the legs, leukorrhea, chronic endometritis, chronic hepatitis, vertigo, and facial flushing
Contraindication	Use with caution during pregnancy

Bupleurum and Peony Combination (Composition)

3.0	*Chai hu*	Bupleurum root	*Bupleuri radix*
1.0	*Bo he*	Field Mint	*Menthae herba*
3.0	*Dang gui*	Tang kuei root	*Angelicae sinensis radix*
3.0	*Shao yao*	Peony	*Paeoniae radix*
3.0	*Bai zhu*	White Atractylodes root	*Atractylodis macrocephalae rhizoma*
3.0	*Fu ling*	Hoelen, Tuckahoe	*Poriae cocos sclerotium*
2.0	*Gan cao*	Licorice root	*Glycyrrhizae uralensis radix*
1.0	*Gan jiang*	Dried ginger rhizome	*Zingiberis officinalis rhizoma*
2.0	*Mu dan pi*	Tree peony root-bark	*Moutan radicis cortex*
2.0	*Zhi zi*	Gardenia fruit	*Gardenia jasminoidis fructus*

Bupleurum and Pueraria Combination

Bupleurum and Pueraria Combination *Chai ge jie ji tang* *(Chai-ko-chieh-chi-tang)*	Bupleurum and Kudzu Decoction to Release the Muscle Layer
Classification	*Fa biao ji:* Surface Relieving, Release Exterior Wind-Heat
Traditional Function	Treats febrile disease by relieving exterior cold and cooling internal heat; relieves pain due to pathogenic factors lodged in the superficial muscle layers
Six Stage Relationship	*Shaoyang-yangming, qi* level
Pulse	Superficial-flooding and rapid
Tongue	Red, dry, thin-yellow coat
Abdomen	Firm
Signs and Symptoms	High fever due to wind-cold or wind-heat, headache, thirst, nasal dryness and nose bleed, general pain, restlessness, painful eye orbits, constipation, and anhidrosis. Hysteria and delirium may occur if fever is too high.
Contraindication	*Yin* deficiency

Bupleurum and Pueraria Combination (Composition)

4.0	*Chai hu*	Bupleurum root	*Bupleuri radix*
3.0	*Huang qin*	Skullcap root, Scute	*Scutellariae baicalensis radix*
3.0	*Shao yao*	Peony	*Paeoniae radix*
5.0	*Shi gao*	Gypsum	*Gypsum fibrosum*
4.0	*Ge gen*	Kudzu root	*Puerariae radix*
2.0	*Bai zhu*	White Atractylodes root	*Atractylodis macrocephalae rhizoma*
2.0	*Qiang huo*	Notopterygium rhizome and root	*Notopterygii rhizoma et radix*
2.0	*Jie geng (ku)*	Balloon flower root, Platycodon	*Platycodi grandiflori radix*
2.0	*Gan cao*	Licorice root	*Glycyrrhizae uralensis radix*
1.0	*Sheng jiang*	Fresh ginger root	*Zingiberis officinalis recens rhizoma*
2.0	*Da zao*	Red date, Jujube fruit	*Ziziphi jujubae fructus*

Bupleurum and Rhubarb Combination

Bupleurum and Rhubarb Combination *Qing yi tang* *(Ching-yi-tang)*	Clear and Augment Decoction
Classification	*Biao li shuang jie ji:* Exterior and Interior Attacking
Traditional Function	Purge heat and promotes bowel movement; regulates qi, and relieves pain
Six Stage Relationship	*Shaoyang-yangming, qi* level
Pulse	Tight, full, and rapid
Tongue	Red with greasy yellow coat
Abdomen	Chest distress with stabbing pain in upper left abdomen
Signs and Symptoms	Fever and chills, constipation, dark colored urine, bitter taste in mouth, and acute pancreatitis
Contraindication	Diarrhea

Bupleurum and Rhubarb Combination (Composition)

5.0	*Chai hu*	Bupleurum root	*Bupleuri radix*
3.0	*Huang qin*	Skullcap root, Scute	*Scutellariae baicalensis radix*
3.0	*Huang lian*	Coptis rhizome	*Coptidis rhizoma*
5.0	*Da huang*	Rhubarb root	*Rhei radix et rhizoma*
3.0	*Yan hu suo*	Corydalis rhizome	*Corydalis rhizome Yanhusuo*
5.0	*Shao yao*	Peony	*Paeoniae radix*
3.0	*Mu xiang*	Saussurea	*Natrium sulphuricum*
3.0	*Mang xiao*	Mirabilite, Glauber's salt	*Mirabilitum*

Bupleurum and Tang Kuei Formula

Bupleurum and Tang Kuei Formula *Xiao yao san* *(Hsiao-yao-san)*	<u>Rambling Powder</u>
Classification	*He jie ji:* Harmonizing
Traditional Function	Treats fever due to stress and heat in the chest with hot palms, soothes the liver, increase spleen and harmonizes the stomach, and promotes *qi* circulation
Six Stage Relationship	*Shaoyang*, blood level
Pulse	Thin, wiry and weak
Tongue	Red, thin-white coat
Abdomen	Distended and painful (mainly around umbilicus)
Signs and Symptoms	Feverish sensation in palms and soles, body ache, dry throat, heaviness in the head, decreased appetite and bitter taste in mouth, insomnia, menstrual irregularity, menopausal disorders, leukorrhea, night sweats, and nervousness in women
Contraindication	*Yang* deficiency

Bupleurum and Tang Kuei Formula (Composition)

3.0	*Chai hu*	Bupleurum root	*Bupleuri radix*
1.0	*Bo he*	Field Mint	*Menthae herba*
3.0	*Dang gui*	Tang kuei root	*Angelicae sinensis radix*
3.0	*Shao yao*	Peony	*Paeoniae radix*
2.0	*Sheng jiang*	Fresh ginger root	*Zingiberis officinalis recens rhizoma*
3.0	*Fu ling*	Hoelen, Tuckahoe	*Poriae cocos sclerotium*
3.0	*Bai zhu*	White Atractylodes root	*Atractylodis macrocephalae rhizoma*
1.5	*Gan cao*	Licorice root	*Glycyrrhizae uralensis radix*

Capillaris Combination

Capillaris Combination *Yin chen hao tang* *(Yin-chen-hao-tang)*	Artemisia Yinchenhao Decoction
Classification	*Li shi ji:* Moisture Dispelling, Clear Damp Heat
Traditional Function	Treats damp-heat in liver and gall bladder, distention and discomfort in the chest and upper abdomen, and jaundice
Six Stage Relationship	*Shaoyang-yangming,* water and blood levels
Pulse	Submerged and strong, slippery-rapid
Tongue	Red, sticky-yellow coat
Abdomen	Abdominal fullness, sensation of discomfort and irritability around the solar plexus region and jaundice
Signs and Symptoms	Jaundice, acute hepatitis, nephritis, nausea, loss of appetite, extreme thirst, vertigo and head sweating, constipation and dark-red scanty urination even after drinking large amounts of fluid, gingivitis, stomatitis, pruritis, uticaria, and uterine bleeding
Contraindication	*Yang* deficiency

Capillaris Combination (Composition)

4.0	*Yin chen hao*	Chinese wormwood	*Artemisiae yinchenhao herba*
3.0	*Zhi zi*	Gardenia fruit	*Gardenia jasminoidis fructus*
1.0	*Da huang*	Rhubarb root	*Rhei radix et rhizoma*

Capillaris and Hoelen Five Formula

Capillaris and Hoelen Five Formula *Yin chen wu ling san* *(Yin-chen-wu-ling-san)*	Artemisia Yinchenhao and Five-Ingredient Powder with Poria
Classification	*Li shi ji:* Moisture Dispelling, Promote Urination and Leech Out Dampness
Traditional Function	Treats liver disorder, jaundice and thirst by dispelling heat and dampness
Six Stage Relationship	*Shaoyang,* water level
Pulse	Floating, slippery, and rapid
Tongue	Red-thick-yellow coat
Abdomen	Soft abdominal wall with water stagnation in stomach
Signs and Symptoms	*Yang*-jaundice, hepatitis, nephritis, sallow complexion, lingering thirst and fever, edema and ascites, and dark-reddish urine
Contraindication	*Yin* deficiency

Capillaris and Hoelen Five Formula (Composition)

6.0	*Yin chen hao*	Chinese wormwood	*Artemisiae yinchenhao herba*
4.0	*Ze xie*	Water plantain rhizome	*Alismatis orientalis rhizoma*
4.5	*Zhu ling*	Polyporus	*Polypori umbellati sclerotium*
4.5	*Bai zhu*	White Atractylodes root	*Atractylodis macrocephalae rhizoma*
4.5	*Fu ling*	Hoelen, Tuckahoe	*Poriae cocos sclerotium*
3.0	*Gui zhi*	Cinnamon twig	*Cinnamomi cassiae ramulus*

Cinnamon Combination

Cinnamon Combination *Gui zhi tang* *(Kuei-chih-tang)*	<u>Cinnamon Twig Decoction</u>
Classification	*Fa biao ji:* Surface Relieving, Release Exterior Cold
Traditional Function	Harmonizes *wei qi* and *ying qi*, relieves external-weak symptoms
Six Stage Relationship	*Taiyang, qi* level
Pulse	Floating and weak
Tongue	Moist, white coat
Abdomen	Spasm in right side
Signs and Symptoms	Fever with spontaneous sweating, general aching, common cold, abdominal pains, headache, dry vomiting, pain under the heart, and a delicate constitution
Contraindication	*Yang* excess

Cinnamon Combination (Composition)

4.0	*Gui zhi*	Cinnamon twig	*Cinnamomi cassiae ramulus*
4.0	*Shao yao*	Peony	*Paeoniae radix*
2.0	*Gan cao*	Licorice root	*Glycyrrhizae uralensis radix*
4.0	*Sheng jiang*	Fresh ginger root	*Zingiberis officinalis recens rhizoma*
4.0	*Da zao*	Red date, Jujube fruit	*Ziziphi jujubae fructus*

Cinnamon, Aconite, and Ginger Combination

Cinnamon, Aconite, and Ginger Combination Gui zhi fu zi tang (Kuei-chi-fu-tzu-tang)	Cinnamon Twig and Prepared Aconite Decoction
Classification	Qu han ji: Chill Dispelling, Release Exterior Cold
Traditional Function	Dispels cold and pain
Six Stage Relationship	Taiyang-shaoyang, water level
Pulse	Floating and weak
Tongue	Pale, thick-white coat
Abdomen	Soft
Signs and Symptoms	Lingering body ache, fever with perspiration, discomfort in the chest, frequent urination, numbness in legs
Contraindication	Yang excess

Cinnamon, Aconite, and Ginger Combination (Composition)

4.0	Gui zhi	Cinnamon twig	Cinnamomi cassiae ramulus
4.0	Shao yao	Peony	Paeoniae radix
2.0	Gan cao	Licorice root	Glycyrrhizae uralensis radix
4.0	Da zao	Red date, Jujube fruit	Ziziphi jujubae fructus
4.0	Gan jiang	Dried ginger rhizome	Zingiberis officinalis rhizoma
0.5-1.0	Fu zi (hei)	Prepared Sichuan aconite root	Lateralis aconiti carmichaeli radix praeparata

Cinnamon and Anemarrhena Combination

Cinnamon and Anemarrhena Combination *Gui zhi shao yao zhi mu tang* *(Kuei-chi-shoa-yao-chih-mu-tang)*	Cinnamon Twig, Peony, and Anemarrhena Decoction
Classification	*Qu feng ji:* Wind Dispelling, Dispel Wind-Dampness
Traditional Function	Dispels cold-wind and damp *Bi* syndrome causing heat stagnation which is worse at night
Six Stage Relationship	*Taiyang, qi* level
Pulse	Slippery, wiry
Tongue	Sticky-white coat
Abdomen	Firm
Signs and Symptoms	Painful hot-swollen joints, paresthesia, muscle atrophy in the legs, emaciation, dyspena and nausea, lower back pain and swollen feet, arthritis, rheumatoid arthritis
Contraindication	Excess heat conditions

Cinnamon and Anemarrhena Combination (Composition)

3.0	*Gui zhi*	Cinnamon twig	*Cinnamomi cassiae ramulus*
3.0	*Shao yao*	Peony	*Paeoniae radix*
3.0	*Ma huang*	Ephedra	*Epherdrae herba*
1.5	*Gan cao*	Licorice root	*Glycyrrhizae uralensis radix*
4.0	*Bai zhu*	White Atractylodes root	*Atractylodis macrocephalae rhizoma*
3.0	*Fang feng*	Siler root	*Ledebouriellae divaricatae radix*
0.5-1.0	*Fu zi (hei)*	Prepared Sichuan aconite root	*Lateralis aconiti carmichaeli radix praeparata*
3.0	*Zhi mu*	Anemarrhena root	*Anemarrhenae asphodeloidis radix*
3.0	*Sheng jiang*	Fresh ginger root	*Zingiberis officinalis recens rhizoma*

Cinnamon and Dragon Bone Combination

Cinnamon and Dragon Bone Combination *Gui zhi jia long gu mu li tang* *(Kuei-chi-chia-lung-ku-mu-li-tang)*	Cinnamon Twig Decoction plus Dragon Bone and Oyster Shell
Classification	*Zhen jing ji:* Sedative, Stabilize the Kidneys
Traditional Function	Harmonizes heart *yin* and kidney *yang*, harmonizes *ying qi* and *wei qi*, induces a calm spirit, delicate constitution with recurrent fever, headache, night sweats, and palpitations
Six Stage Relationship	*Shaoyin, qi* level
Pulse	Slow, big and weak
Tongue	Pale
Abdomen	Spasms in lower abdomen, palpitations around the umbilicus
Signs and Symptoms	Palpitations, nervousness, insomnia, night sweats, enuresis, anxiety and fright, headache, dizziness, nocturnal emissions and premature ejaculation, nervous exhaustion due to sexual excess, excitability, and fatigue
Contraindication	*Yang* excess

Cinnamon and Dragon Bone Combination (Composition)

4.0	*Gui zhi*	Cinnamon twig	*Cinnamomi cassiae ramulus*
4.0	*Shao yao*	Peony	*Paeoniae radix*
4.0	*Da zao*	Red date, Jujube fruit	*Ziziphi jujubae fructus*
4.0	*Sheng jiang*	Fresh ginger root	*Zingiberis officinalis recens rhizoma*
2.0	*Gan cao*	Licorice root	*Glycyrrhizae uralensis radix*
3.0	*Long gu*	Dragon bone	*Os draconis*
3.0	*Mu li*	Oyster shell	*Ostreae concha*

Cinnamon and Hoelen Formula

Cinnamon and Hoelen Formula *Gui zhi fu ling wan* *(Kuei-chih-fu-ling-wan)*	Cinnamon Twig and Poria Pill
Classification	*Li xie ji:* Blood Regulating, Warm the Menses and Dispel Blood Stasis
Traditional Function	Treats gynecological, skin, and neuropathy disorders related to blood stagnation
Six Stage Relationship	*Shaoyang,* blood level
Pulse	Tight or deep and slow
Tongue	Purple with a sticky coat
Abdomen	Lower abdominal fullness and pain (mainly on the left side of umbilicus), masses painful upon pressure
Signs and Symptoms	Cold feet and signs of blood stagnation in face and lips, dizziness, headache, lumps in lower abdomen, black spots, menstrual irregularity, and nervousness
Contraindication	Pregnancy

Cinnamon and Hoelen Formula (Composition)

4.0	*Gui zhi*	Cinnamon twig	*Cinnamomi cassiae ramulus*
4.0	*Mu dan pi*	Tree peony root-bark	*Moutan radicis cortex*
4.0	*Shao yao*	Peony	*Paeoniae radix*
4.0	*Tao ren*	Peach kernel	*Persicae semen*
4.0	*Fu ling*	Hoelen, Tuckahoe	*Poriae cocos sclerotium*

Cinnamon Ma-huang Combination

Cinnamon Ma-huang Combination *Gui zhi ma huang ge ban tang* *(Kuei-chih-ma-huang-ko-pan-tang)*	Combined Cinnamon Twig and Ephedra
Classification	*Fa biao ji:* Surface Relieving, Release Exterior Cold
Traditional Function	Relieves exterior-strong symptoms, promote lung qi circulation
Six Stage Relationship	*Taiyang, qi* level
Pulse	Floating weak
Tongue	Red tip, white coat
Abdomen	Firm
Signs and Symptoms	Fever with mild chills, facial reddening, itching skin, and headache
Contraindication	Constipation

Cinnamon Ma-huang Combination (Composition)

3.5	*Gui zhi*	Cinnamon twig	*Cinnamomi cassiae ramulus*
2.0	*Shao yao*	Peony	*Paeoniae radix*
2.0	*Sheng jiang*	Fresh ginger root	*Zingiberis officinalis recens rhizoma*
2.0	*Da zao*	Red date, Jujube fruit	*Ziziphi jujubae fructus*
2.0	*Gan cao*	Licorice root	*Glycyrrhizae uralensis radix*
2.0	*Ma huang*	Ephedra	*Epherdrae herba*
2.5	*Xing ren*	Apricot seed	*Pruni armeniacae semen*

Cinnamon, Magnolia, and Apricot Seed Combination

Cinnamon, Magnolia, and Apricot Seed Combination *Gui zhi jia hou pu xing ren tang* *(Kuei-chih-chia-hou-pu-hsing-jen-tang)*	Cinnamon Twig Decoction plus Magnolia Bark and Apricot Kernel
Classification	*Fa biao ji:* Surface Relieving, Release Exterior Cold
Traditional Function	Relieves exterior, suppresses cough and relaxes breathing
Six Stage Relationship	*Taiyang, qi* level
Pulse	Floating and tight
Tongue	Light red
Abdomen	Firm
Signs and Symptoms	Cough, asthma, spontaneous sweating, headache, worse with exposure to wind and cold
Contraindication	*Yang* excess

Cinnamon, Magnolia, and Apricot Seed Combination (Composition)

4.0	*Gui zhi*	Cinnamon twig	*Cinnamomi cassiae ramulus*
4.0	*Shao yao*	Peony	*Paeoniae radix*
4.0	*Sheng jiang*	Fresh ginger root	*Zingiberis officinalis recens rhizoma*
4.0	*Da zao*	Red date, Jujube fruit	*Ziziphi jujubae fructus*
4.0	*Gan cao*	Licorice root	*Glycyrrhizae uralensis radix*
1.0	*Hou po*	Magnolia bark	*Magnoliae officinalis cortex*
4.0	*Xing ren*	Apricot seed	*Pruni armeniacae semen*

Cinnamon and Peony Combination

Cinnamon and Peony Combination *Gui zhi jia shao yao tang* *(Kuai-chih-chia-shao-yao-tang)*	Cinnamon Twig Decoction Plus Peony
Classification	*Fa biao ji:* Surface Relieving, Release Exterior Cold
Traditional Function	Dispel cold, relieves muscle spasms and pain, and warms the middle *San Jiao*
Six Stage Relationship	*Taiyang, qi* level
Pulse	Floating-fast pulse
Tongue	Thin-white tongue coating
Abdomen	Congested
Signs and Symptoms	Intermittent abdominal pain and fullness, hypochondriac pain (right side), headache, fever, mild shoulder stiffness, mild diarrhea, enteritis, appendicitis, peritonitis
Contraindication	Constipation

Cinnamon and Peony Combination (Composition)

4.0	*Gui zhi*	Cinnamon twig	*Cinnamomi cassiae ramulus*
6.0	*Shao yao*	Peony	*Paeoniae radix*
4.0	*Sheng jiang*	Fresh ginger root	*Zingiberis officinalis recens rhizoma*
4.0	*Da zao*	Red date, Jujube fruit	*Ziziphi jujubae fructus*
4.0	*Gan cao*	Licorice root	*Glycyrrhizae uralensis radix*

Cinnamon and Pueraria Combination

Cinnamon and Pueraria Combination *Gui zhi jia ge gen tang or* *Xiao ge gen tang* *(Kuei-chih-chia-ko-ken-tang)* *or (Hsiao-ko-ken-tang)*	Cinnamon Twig Decoction plus Kudzu
Classification	*Fa biao ji:* Surface Relieving, Release Exterior Cold
Traditional Function	Dispels wind-cold symptoms and relaxes muscles
Six Stage Relationship	*Taiyang-qi* level
Pulse	Floating, tight
Tongue	Red, thin white coat
Abdomen	Firm
Signs and Symptoms	Initial stage of febrile diseases, stiffness and pain in the neck and upper back, spontaneous sweating and chills, and headache
Contraindication	*Yang* excess

Cinnamon and Pueraria Combination (Composition)

6.0	*Ge gen*	Kudzu root	*Puerariae radix*
4.0	*Gui zhi*	Cinnamon twig	*Cinnamomi cassiae ramulus*
4.0	*Shao yao*	Peony	*Paeoniae radix*
4.0	*Sheng jiang*	Fresh ginger root	*Zingiberis officinalis recens rhizoma*
4.0	*Da zao*	Red date, Jujube fruit	*Ziziphi jujubae fructus*
2.0	*Gan cao*	Licorice root	*Glycyrrhizae uralensis radix*

Coix Combination

Coix Combination *Yi yi ren tang* (*I-yi-jen-tang*)	Coix Decoction
Classification	*Li shi ji:* Moisture Dispelling, Promote Urination and Leech Out Dampness
Traditional Function	Dispel wind-cold and damp-cold, invigorate blood, and relieves numbness and pain
Six Stage Relationship	*Taiyang/Jueyin,* water and blood levels
Pulse	Tight or slippery
Tongue	Red or purple, glossy coat
Abdomen	Swollen and painful, with spasms
Signs and Symptoms	Painful and swollen joints (worst in cold weather), pain and spasms in limbs, lingering feverish sensation in limbs, chronic rheumatoid arthritis, impaired movement in legs, and cysts on fleshy areas of the body
Contraindication	Excess *yang*

Coix Combination (Composition)

4.0	*Ma huang*	Ephedra	*Epherdrae herba*
3.0	*Gui zhi*	Cinnamon twig	*Cinnamomi cassiae ramulus*
4.0	*Bai zhu*	White Atractylodes root	*Atractylodis macrocephalae rhizoma*
4.0	*Dang gui*	Tang kuei root	*Angelicae sinensis radix*
3.0	*Shao yao*	Peony	*Paeoniae radix*
8.0	*Yi yi ren*	Job's tears, Coxis	*Coicis lachryma-jobi*
2.0	*Gan cao*	Licorice root	*Glycyrrhizae uralensis radix*

Coptis Combination

Coptis Combination *Huang lien tang* *(Huang-Lien-tang)*	Coptis Decoction
Classification	*He jie ji:* Harmonizing, Harmonize the Stomach and Intestines
Traditional Function	Harmonizes spleen and stomach, clears heat in upper *jiao* and cold stagnation in middle *jiao*
Six Stage Relationship	*Shaoyang, qi* level
Pulse	Floating and full in *cun* position; and submerged in *guan* and *chi* positions
Tongue	Red, sticky white-yellow coat
Abdomen	Upper abdominal pain
Signs and Symptoms	Fever in the chest with a sensation of pressure and stagnancy in the stomach, loss of appetite, nausea, vomiting, fetid breath, irregular bowel movements, and acute food poisoning
Contraindication	*Yin* deficiency

Coptis Combination (Composition)

3.0	*Huang lian*	Coptis rhizome	*Coptidis rhizoma*
3.0	*Gan jiang*	Dried ginger rhizome	*Zingiberis officinalis rhizoma*
3.0	*Gui zhi*	Cinnamon twig	*Cinnamomi cassiae ramulus*
6.0	*Ban xia (fa)*	Pinellia rhizome	*Pinelliae ternatae rhizoma*
3.0	*Ren shen*	Ginseng root	*Ginseng radix*
3.0	*Gan cao*	Licorice root	*Glycyrrhizae uralensis radix*
3.0	*Da zao*	Red date, Jujube fruit	*Ziziphi jujubae fructus*

Coptis and Rhubarb Combination

Coptis and Rhubarb Combination *San huang xie xin tang* *(San-huang-hsieh-his- tang)*	Three-Yellow Decoction to Drain the Epigastrium
Classification	*Qing re xie huo ji:* Fire Purging
Traditional Function	Clears internal heat from *yangming* and stops bleeding due to heat
Six Stage Relationship	*Yangming, qi* and blood levels
Pulse	Flooding and rapid
Tongue	Dark red, yellow coat
Abdomen	Distended, hard, and tense
Signs and Symptoms	Habitual constipation, dysentery, liver disorders, hypertension, intestinal bleeding, hematuria, uterine bleeding, hemoptysis, facial flushing, and a sensation of distention and stagnancy in the stomach region
Contraindication	Pregnancy, persons with a weak-minute pulse and anemia

Coptis and Rhubarb Combination (Composition)

1.0	*Da huang*	Rhubarb root	*Rhei radix et rhizoma*
1.0	*Huang lian*	Coptis rhizome	*Coptidis rhizoma*
1.0	*Huang qin*	Skullcap root, Scute	*Scutellariae baicalensis radix*

Coptis and Scute Combination

Coptis and Scute Combination *Huang lian jie du tang* *(Huang-lien-chieh-tu-tang)*	Coptis Decoction to Relieve Toxicity
Classification	*Qin re xie hue ji:* Fire Purging, Clear Heat and Relieve Toxicity
Traditional Function	Purge fire from the *yangming*, arrests bleeding and relieves irritability due to heat
Six Stage Relationship	*Yangming, qi* and blood levels
Pulse	Sunken and forceful
Tongue	Red, yellow coat
Abdomen	Tight
Signs and Symptoms	Fever, facial reddening, black stools resembling tar, bleeding disorders (due to true heat), insomnia, discomfort in the chest, and sensation of resistance beneath the heart
Contraindication	*Yin* deficiency

Coptis and Scute Combination (Composition)

1.5	*Huang lian*	Coptis rhizome	*Coptidis rhizoma*
3.0	*Huang qin*	Skullcap root, Scute	*Scutellariae baicalensis radix*
1.5	*Huang bai*	Amur cork-tree bark	*Phellodendri cortex*

Cyperus and Perilla Formula

Cyperus and Perilla Formula *Xiang su san* *(Hsiang-su-san)*	<u>Cyperus and Perilla Leaf Decoction</u>
Classification	*Fa biao ji:* Surface Relieving
Traditional Function	Harmonizes external wind cold symptoms and *qi* stagnation in the middle *jiao*
Six Stage Relationship	*Shaoyang, qi* level
Pulse	Submerged and tight, or superficial and tight
Tongue	Thin-white coat
Abdomen	Obstructed and distended sensation in the upper-middle region with pain
Signs and Symptoms	Common cold with gastrointestinal weakness, headache, stiff shoulders, nausea and vomiting, heavy-headedness, fish poisoning and urticaria
Contraindication	*Yang* excess

Cyperus and Perilla Formula (Composition)

3.5	*Xiang fu zi*	Nut-grass rhizome, Cyperus	*Cyperi rotundi rhizoma*
1.5	*Zi su ye*	Perilla leaf	*Perillae frutescentis folium*
3.0	*Chen pi*	Tangerine peel	*Citri reticulatae pericarpium*
1.0	*Sheng jiang*	Fresh ginger root	*Zingiberis officinalis recens rhizoma*
1.0	*Gan cao*	Licorice root	*Glycyrrhizae uralensis radix*

Evodia Combination

Evodia Combination *Wu zhu yu tang* *(Wu-chu-yu-tang)*	Evodia Decoction
Classification	*Qu han ji*: Chill Dispelling, Warm the Middle and Dispel Cold
Traditional Function	Dispels cold in the liver, spleen, and stomach, supplements spleen qi
Six Stage Relationship	*Shaoyang, qi* level
Pulse	Wiry and slow
Tongue	Pale, purplish, moist-white coat
Abdomen	Firm, water sounds in stomach upon palpating
Signs and Symptoms	Vomiting (morning sickness), excessive salivation, sub cardiac distention with cold limbs, acute vomiting and diarrhea, and discomfort in the chest with a sensation of heaviness below the heart
Contraindication	*Yang* excess

Evodia Combination (Composition)

4.0	*Wu zhu yu*	Evodia fruit	*Evodiae rutaecarpae fructus*
6.0	*Sheng jiang*	Fresh ginger root	*Zingiberis officinalis recens rhizoma*
3.0	*Ren shen*	Ginseng root	*Ginseng radix*
3.0	*Da zao*	Red date, Jujube fruit	*Ziziphi jujubae fructus*

Gentiana Combination

Gentiana Combination *Long dan xie gan tang (Lung-tan-hsieh-kan-tang)*	Gentiana Longdan Cao Decoction to Drain the Liver
Classification	*Qing re xie ji:* Fire Purging, Clear Heat form the Organs
Traditional Function	Clears damp-heat and liver fire
Six Stage Relationship	*Yangming*, blood level
Pulse	Wiry, slippery, and rapid
Tongue	Red, thick-yellow coat
Abdomen	Painful and swollen lower section, hypersensitivity on the outer sides
Signs and Symptoms	Dark-colored and turbid urine, swelling and itching in the genital region, bloodshot eyes, deafness, vaginal inflammation
Contraindication	*Yin* deficiency

Gentiana Combination (Composition)

1.0	*Long dan cao*	Gentian root	*Gentianae longdancao radix*
3.0	*Ze xie*	Water plantain rhizome	*Alismatis orientalis rhizoma*
5.0	*Mu tong*	Akebia stem	*Mutong caulis*
3.0	*Che qian zi*	Plantago seed	*Plantaginis semen*
5.0	*Dang gui*	Tang kuei root	*Angelicae sinensis radix*
5.0	*Sheng di huang*	Fresh rehmannia root, Chinese foxglove root	*Rehmanniae glutinosae radix*
1.0	*Zhi zi*	Gardenia fruit	*Gardenia jasminoidis fructus*
3.0	*Huang qin*	Skullcap root, Scute	*Scutellariae baicalensis radix*
1.0	*Gan cao*	Licorice root	*Glycyrrhizae uralensis radix*

Ginseng and Astragalus Combination

Ginseng and Astragalus Combination *Bu zhong yi qi tang* *(Pu-chung-i-chi-tang)*	Tonify the Middle and Augment and Qi Decoction
Classification	*Bu yi ji:* Tonic and Replenishing, Tonify the Qi
Traditional Function	Increase qi, supplements spleen and stomach
Six Stage Relationship	*Taiyin qi* level
Pulse	Weak
Tongue	Pale, swollen, thin-white coat
Abdomen	Weak with palpitations at the umbilicus
Signs and Symptoms	Fatigue, organ prolapse, loss of appetite and weight, night sweats, spontaneous sweats, weak gastrointestinal tract
Contraindication	*Yang* excess

Ginseng and Astragalus Combination (Composition)

4.0	*Huang qi*	Astragalus Root, Yellow milk-vetch root	*Astragali membranaceus radix*
4.0	*Ren shen*	Ginseng root	*Ginseng radix*
1.5	*Gan cao*	Licorice root	*Glycyrrhizae uralensis radix*
4.0	*Bai zhu*	White Atractylodes root	*Atractylodis macrocephalae rhizoma*
2.0	*Chen pi*	Tangerine peel	*Citri reticulatae pericarpium*
3.0	*Dang gui*	Tang kuei root	*Angelicae sinensis radix*
2.0	*Chai hu*	Bupleurum root	*Bupleuri radix*
1.0	*Sheng ma*	Bugbane, Black Cohosh Rhizome, Cimicifuga	*Cimicifugae rhizoma*
2.0	*Sheng jiang*	Fresh ginger root	*Zingiberis officinalis recens rhizoma*
2.0	*Da zao*	Red date, Jujube fruit	*Ziziphi jujubae fructus*

Ginseng and Gypsum Combination

Ginseng and Gypsum Combination *Bai hu jia ren shen tang* *(Pai-hu-chia-jen-sheng-tang)*	White Tiger plus Ginseng Decoction
Classification	*Qing re xie huo ji:* Fire Purging, Clear Heat form the Qi Level
Traditional Function	Clears heat, increase body fluids and relieves thirst, calm the spirit
Six Stage Relationship	*Yangming, qi* level
Pulse	Flooding, rapid, weak or strong
Tongue	Red, dry-yellow coat
Abdomen	Fullness, soft
Signs and Symptoms	Constipation, fever with chills in the back, heaviness and pain in the limbs, frequent urination, discomfort and irritability in the chest, thirst, dry-mouth and tongue
Contraindication	*Yin* excess

Ginseng and Gypsum Combination (Composition)

5.0	*Zhi mu*	Anemarrhena root	*Anemarrhenae asphodeloidis radix*
15.0	*Shi gao*	Gypsum	*Gypsum fibrosum*
10.0	*Jing mi*	Rice grain	*Oryzae sativae semen*
2.0	*Gan cao*	Licorice root	*Glycyrrhizae uralensis radix*
3.0	*Ren shen*	Ginseng root	*Ginseng radix*

Ginseng and Zanthoxylum Combination

Ginseng and Zanthoxylum Combination *Li Zhong An Hui Tang* *(Li-Chung-An-Huei-Tang)*	Regulate the Middle and Calm Roundworms Decoction
Classification	*Qu Chong Ji:* Anthelmintic
Traditional Function	Eliminates parasites, warms the interior, regulates stomach, and spleen
Six Stage Relationship	*Jueyin, qi* and water level
Pulse	Weak
Tongue	Pale, thin-white coating
Abdomen	Weak and painful with borborygmus
Signs and Symptoms	Cold limbs, gastrointestinal weakness, ascariasis, watery diarrhea, abdominal pain, worms in vomit or stools, and clear and profuse urine
Contraindication	*Yang* excess

Ginseng and Zanthoxylum Combination (Composition)

1.5	*Ren shen*	Ginseng root	*Ginseng radix*
1.5	*Gan jiang*	Ginger (dried)	*Zingiberis siccatum rhizoma*
5.0	*Bai zhu*	Atractylodes (white)	*Atractylodis rhizoma*
6.0	*Fu ling*	Hoelen	*Poria*
1.5	*Shan jiao*	Zanthoxylum	*Zanthoxyli fructus*
2.0	*Wu mei*	Mume	*Mume fructus*

Ginseng and Zizyphus Combination

Ginseng and Zizyphus Combination *Tien wang bu xin dan* *(Tien-wang-pu-hsin-tan)*	Emperors of Heaven's Special Pill to Tonify the Heart
Classification	*Bu yi ji:* Tonic and Replenishing, Nourish the Heart and Calm the Spirit
Traditional Function	Nourishes heart *yin*, supplements blood, and calms the spirit
Six Stage Relationship	*Shaoyin*, blood level
Pulse	Theady, weak, and rapid
Tongue	Red, without coat
Abdomen	Weak and flaccid, strong pulsation of the abdominal aorta
Signs and Symptoms	Palpitations with emotional instability, profuse sweating, absentmindedness, lingering fever, constipation or watery diarrhea
Contraindication	Patients with gastrointestinal weakness and excessive sputum
Contraindication	*Yang* excess

Ginseng and Zizyphus Combination (Composition)

1.2	*Sheng di huang*	Fresh rehmannia root, Chinese foxglove root	*Rehmanniae glutinosae radix*
1.2	*Xuan shen*	Scophularia root, Figwort root	*Scrophulariae radix*
1.2	*Tian men dong*	Chinese asparagus tuber	*Asparagi cochinchinensis tuber*
1.2	*Dang gui*	Tang kuei root	*Angelicae sinensis radix*
1.2	*Mai men dong*	Ophiopogon tuber, Creeping lily-turf tuber	*Ophiopogonis japonici tuber*
1.2	*Dang gui*	Tang kuei root	*Angelicae sinensis radix*
1.2	*Dan shen*	Salvia root	*Salviae miltiorrhizae radix*
1.2	*Ren shen*	Ginseng root	*Ginseng radix*
1.2	*Fu ling*	Hoelen, Tuckahoe	*Poriae cocos sclerotium*

1.2	*Wu zhu yu*	Evodia fruit	*Evodiae rutaecarpae fructus*
1.2	*Bai zi ren*	Biota seed	*Biotae orientalis semen*
1.2	*Suan zao ren*	Zizyphus seed, Sour jujube	*Zizyphi spinosae semen*
1.2	*Yuan Zhi*	Polygala Root	*Radix Polygalae Tenuifoliae*
1.2	*Zhu sha*	Kansui spurge root	*Euphorbiae kansui radix*
1.2	*Shi chang pu*	Acorus, Sweetflag rhizome	*Acori graminei rhizoma*
1.2	*Huang lian*	Coptis rhizome	*Coptidis rhizoma*

Gypsum Combination

Gypsum Combination *Bai hu tang* *(Pai-hu-tang)*	<u>White Tiger Decoction</u>
Classification	*Qing re xie huo ji:* Fire Purging, Clear Heat from Qi Level
Traditional Function	Dispels wind and toxic heat and nourishes yin
Six Stage Relationship	*Shaoyang-yangming, qi* level
Pulse	Big and strong, floating and slippery
Tongue	Red, white coat
Abdomen	Full and tight
Signs and Symptoms	High fever, extreme thirst, dry coarse skin, spontaneous sweating, aversion to heat, excessive urination, incontinence, and skin disorders due to toxic heat
Contraindication	Pale complexion and sweating, fever without thirst, and chills without sweating

Gypsum Combination (Composition)

2.0	*Da huang*	Rhubarb root	*Rhei radix et rhizoma*
2.0	*Zhi shi*	Immature bitter orange fruit	*Citri seu ponciri immaturus fructus*
3.0	*Hou po*	Magnolia bark	*Magnoliae officinalis cortex*

Gypsum and Apricot Seed Combination

Gypsum and Apricot Seed Combination *Wu hu tang* *(Wu-hu-Tang)*	<u>Gypsum and Apricot Seed Decoction</u>
Classification	*Fa biao ji:* Surface Relieving
Traditional Function	Clears lung heat, relieves cough and asthma and external symptoms
Six Stage Relationship	*Taiyang, qi* level
Pulse	Floating and strong
Tongue	Red, dry-yellow coat
Abdomen	Firm
Signs and Symptoms	Bronchial asthma, slight sweating, dry cough accompanied by sore throat, and thirst for cold water
Contraindication	*Yin* excess

Gypsum and Apricot Seed Combination (Composition)

10.0	*Shi gao*	Gypsum	*Gypsum fibrosum*
4.0	*Ma huang*	Ephedra	*Epherdrae herba*
4.0	*Xing ren*	Apricot seed	*Pruni armeniacae semen*
2.0	*Gan cao*	Licorice root	*Glycyrrhizae uralensis radix*

Gypsum, Coptis, and Scute Combination

Gypsum, Coptis, and Scute Combination *San huang shi gao tang* *(San-huang-shih-kao-tang)*	Three Yellows with Gypsum Decoction
Classification	*Biao li shuang jie j:* Exterior and Interior Attacking
Traditional Function	Treats toxic heat, promotes sweating and clears skin eruptions
Six Stage Relationship	*Taiyang-shaoyang, qi* and blood levels
Pulse	Big and rapid
Tongue	Red
Abdomen	Firm
Signs and Symptoms	High fever, red face, dry mouth and nasal passage, nosebleeds, insomnia, delirium, hemorrhage due to inflammation
Contraindication	*Yin* excess

Gypsum, Coptis, and Scute Combination (Composition)

3.0	*Huang qin*	Skullcap root, Scute	*Scutellariae baicalensis radix*
1.5	*Huang lian*	Coptis rhizome	*Coptidis rhizoma*
1.5	*Huang bai*	Amur cork-tree bark	*Phellodendri cortex*
2.0	*Zhi shi*	Immature bitter orange fruit	*Citri seu ponciri immaturus fructus*
10.0	*Shi gao*	Gypsum	*Gypsum fibrosum*
3.0	*Ma huang*	Ephedra	*Epherdrae herba*
2.0	*Dan dou chi*	Soybean prepared	*Sojae praeparatum semen*
1.0	*Sheng jiang*	Fresh ginger root	*Zingiberis officinalis recens rhizoma*
1.0	*Da zao*	Red date, Jujube fruit	*Ziziphi jujubae fructus*
1.0	*Cha ye*	Tea	*Camelliae folium*

Hoelen Five Herb Combination

Hoelen Five Herb Combination *Wu Ling san* *(Wu-ling-san)*	Five Ingredient Powder with Poria
Classification	*Li shi ji:* Moisture Dispelling, Promote Urination and Leech Out Dampness
Traditional Function	Harmonizes water metabolism, promotes yang, and dispels dampness
Six Stage Relationship	*Shaoyang,* water level
Pulse	Floating and rapid, submerged and soft
Tongue	Red, thick coat
Abdomen	Soft and edematous, painful
Signs and Symptoms	Vomiting after intake of fluids, vomiting with diarrhea, vertigo, anxiety, and palpitations, motion sickness, toxemia during pregnancy, and excessive salivation
Contraindication	*Yin* deficiency

Hoelen Five Herb Combination (Composition)

6.0	*Ze xie*	Water plantain rhizome	*Alismatis orientalis rhizoma*
4.5	*Zhu ling*	Polyporus	*Polypori umbellati sclerotium*
4.5	*Fu ling*	Hoelen, Tuckahoe	*Poriae cocos sclerotium*
4.5	*Bai zhu*	White Atractylodes root	*Atractylodis macrocephalae rhizoma*
3.0	*Gui zhi*	Cinnamon twig	*Cinnamomi cassiae ramulus*

Kaolin and Oryza Combination

Kaolin and Oryza Combination *Tao hua tang* *(Tao-hua-tang)*	Kaolin and Oryza Decoction
Classification	*Shou se ji:* Astringent
Traditional Function	Treats a delicate constitution, warms and nourishes the stomach and spleen, dispels internal chills, prevents bleeding, and regulates blood
Six Stage Relationship	*Shaoyin,* blood level
Pulse	Deep, slow, and thready
Tongue	Pale, thick-white coat
Abdomen	Fullness, distention, and painful
Signs and Symptoms	General weakness, cold extremities, diarrhea with pustulent bloody stool, decreased urination, absence of fever and tenesmus
Contraindication	*Yang* excess

Kaolin and Oryza Combination (Composition)

6.0	*Chi shi zhi*	Kaolin	*Halloysitum rubrum*
1.5	*Gan jiang*	Dried ginger rhizome	*Zingiberis officinalis rhizoma*
8.0	*Jing mi*	Rice grain	*Oryzae sativae semen*

Kaolin and Oryza Combination

Kaolin and Oryza Combination *Tong mai si ni tang* *(Tung-mo-szu-ni-tang)*	<u>Unblock the Pulse for Frigid Extremities</u>
Classification	*Qu han j:* Chill Dispelling, Rescue Devastated Yang
Traditional Function	Increase depleted *yang* and restores the pulse
Six Stage Relationship	*Jueyin, qi* level
Pulse	Very weak and slow
Tongue	Pale
Abdomen	Weak with sucussion sounds
Signs and Symptoms	Cold limbs, heavy pressure sensation below the heart, fatigue, internal chills and external fever
Contraindication	*Yang* excess

Licorice, Aconite, and Ginger Pulse Combination (Composition)

0.5-1.0	*Fu zi (hei)*	Prepared Sichuan aconite root	*Lateralis aconiti carmichaeli radix praeparata*
4.0	*Gan jiang*	Dried ginger rhizome	*Zingiberis officinalis rhizoma*
3.0	*Gan cao*	Licorice root	*Glycyrrhizae uralensis radix*

Licorice and Ginger Combination

Licorice and Ginger Combination *Gan cao gan jiang tang* *(Kan-tsao-kan-chiang-tang)*	Licorice and Ginger Decoction
Classification	*Qu han ji:* Chill Dispelling, Warm the Middle and Dispel Cold
Traditional Function	Increase *yang*, dispels cold, increase spleen and stomach *qi*
Six Stage Relationship	*Jueyin, qi* level
Pulse	Weak
Tongue	Pale and moist
Abdomen	Soft and weak
Signs and Symptoms	Weak and debilitated constitution, cold limbs and dizziness, frequent urination, *yang qi* deficiency due to excessive use of diaphoretics
Contraindication	*Yang* excess

Licorice and Ginger Combination (Composition)

4.0	*Gan cao*	Licorice root	*Glycyrrhizae uralensis radix*
2.0	*Gan jiang*	Dried ginger rhizome	*Zingiberis officinalis rhizoma*

Ma-huang Combination

Ma-huang Combination *Ma huang tang* (Ma-huang-tang)	Ephedra Decoction
Classification	*Fa biao ji:* Surface Relieving, Release Early-Stage Exterior
Traditional Function	Induces sweating, promotes lung qi circulation
Six Stage Relationship	*Taiyang, qi* level
Pulse	Floating and tight
Tongue	Red, thin-white coat
Abdomen	Firm
Signs and Symptoms	Fever without sweating caused by a cold-wind invasion, general aching and joint pain, lower back pain, headaches, distention in the chest
Contraindication	*Yin* deficiency

Ma-huang Combination (Composition)

5.0	*Xing ren*	Apricot seed	*Pruni armeniacae semen*
5.0	*Ma huang*	Ephedra	*Epherdrae herba*
4.0	*Gui zhi*	Cinnamon twig	*Cinnamomi cassiae ramulus*
1.5	*Gan cao*	Licorice root	*Glycyrrhizae uralensis radix*

Ma-huang, Aconite, and Asarum Combination

Ma-huang, Aconite, and Asarum Combination or Ma-Huang and Asarum Combination *Ma huang fu zi xi xin tang* (*Ma-huang-fu-tzu-hsi-hsin-tang*)	Ephedra, Asarum, and Prepared Aconite Decoction
Classification	*Fa biao ji:* Surface Relieving
Traditional Function	Dispels chill and restores *yang*
Six Stage Relationship	*Jueyin, qi* level
Pulse	Submerged, thin, and weak
Tongue	Pale, thin-white coat
Abdomen	Weak with water stagnation below the heart
Signs and Symptoms	General aching, lassitude and exhaustion, Frequent or painful urination, cold limbs, pallor facial complexion, edema, chills in the back and head
Contraindication	*Yang* deficiency

Ma-huang, Aconite, and Asarum Combination (Composition)

4.0	*Ma huang*	Ephedra	*Epherdrae herba*
3.0	*Xi xin*	Asarum, Chinese wild ginger	*Asari herba radice*
0.5-1.0	*Fu zi (hei)*	Prepared Sichuan aconite root	*Lateralis aconiti carmichaeli radix praeparata*

Ma-huang, Aconite, and Licorice Combination

Ma-huang, Aconite, and Licorice Combination *Ma huang fu zi gan cao tang* *(Ma-huang-fu-tzu-kan-tsao-tang)*	Ephedra, Prepared Aconite, and Licorice Decoction
Classification	*Fa biao ji:* Surface Relieving, Release Exterior with Interior Deficiency
Traditional Function	Dispels chill and restores *yang*
Six Stage Relationship	*Taiyang-Jueyin, qi* level
Pulse	Submerged and thin
Tongue	Pale, thin-white coat
Abdomen	Weak
Signs and Symptoms	Cold limbs, chills and mild fever, fatigue, general mild aching and edema, cough and shortness of breath, sensation of discomfort in the heart
Contraindication	*Yang* excess

Ma-huang, Aconite, and Licorice Combination (Composition)

3.0	*Ma huang*	Ephedra	*Epherdrae herba*
0.5-1.0	*Fu zi (hei)*	Prepared Sichuan aconite root	*Lateralis aconiti carmichaeli radix praeparata*
3.0	*Gan cao*	Licorice root	*Glycyrrhizae uralensis radix*

Ma-huang and Apricot Seed Combination

Ma-huang and Apricot Seed Combination *Ma xing gan shi tang* *(Ma-hsing-kan-shih-tang)*	Ephedra, Apricot Kernel, Gypsum, and Licorice Decoction
Classification	*Fa baio ji:* Surface Relieving, Clear Heat form the Organs
Traditional Function	Treats lung heat caused by cold-wind with external symptoms, relieves cough and asthma, improves lung *qi* circulation
Six Stage Relationship	*Taiyang, qi* level
Pulse	Floating, tight, and rapid
Tongue	Red, thin-white coat
Abdomen	Firm
Signs and Symptoms	Cough and difficult breathing, thirst, swelling of the face and eyes, spontaneous sweating
Contraindication	*Yin* deficiency

Ma-huang and Apricot Seed Combination (Composition)

10.0	*Shi gao*	Gypsum	*Gypsum fibrosum*
4.0	*Ma huang*	Ephedra	*Epherdrae herba*
4.0	*Xing ren*	Apricot seed	*Pruni armeniacae semen*
2.0	*Gan cao*	Licorice root	*Glycyrrhizae uralensis radix*

Ma-huang and Asarum Combination

Ma-huang and Asarum Combination *Ma huang fu zi xi xin tang* *(Ma-huang-fu-tzu-hsi-hsin-tang)*	<u>Ephedra, Asarum, and Prepared Aconite Decoction</u>
Classification	*Fa biao ji:* Surface Relieving, Release Exterior with Interior Deficiency
Traditional Function	Dispels chill and restores yang
Six Stage Relationship	*Jueyin, qi* level
Pulse	Submerged and thready
Tongue	Pale, white coat
Abdomen	Soft distended, and weak
Signs and Symptoms	Weak or elderly patients, cold limbs, chills and mild fever, expectoration of thin water-like sputum, lassitude, cough, and bronchial asthma
Contraindication	*Yin* deficiency

Ma-huang and Asarum Combination (Composition)

4.0	*Ma huang*	Ephedra	*Epherdrae herba*
3.0	*Xi xin*	Asarum, Chinese wild ginger	*Asari herba radice*
0.5-1.0	*Fu zi (hei)*	Prepared Sichuan aconite root	*Lateralis aconiti carmichaeli radix praeparata*

Ma-huang and Atractylodes Combination

Ma-huang and Atractylodes Combination *Ma huang jia shu tang (Ma-huang-chia-chu-tang)*	Ephedra Decoction plus Atractylodis
Classification	*Fa biao ji:* Surface Relieving, Release Exterior Cold
Traditional Function	Treats surface-fever-firm symptoms, promotes lung qi circulation, reduces edema
Six Stage Relationship	*Taiyang*, water level
Pulse	Floating, moderate-tight
Tongue	Red, moist-white coat
Abdomen	Firm
Signs and Symptoms	Body ache, fever, chills and anhidrosis, edema and decreased urination, arthralgia, headache due to carbon monoxide or other toxic gas poisoning
Contraindication	*Yin* deficiency

Ma-huang and Atractylodes Combination (Composition)

4.0	*Gui zhi*	Cinnamon twig	*Cinnamomi cassiae ramulus*
5.0	*Ma huang*	Ephedra	*Epherdrae herba*
5.0	*Xing ren*	Apricot seed	*Pruni armeniacae semen*
5.0	*Bai zhu*	White Atractylodes root	*Atractylodis macrocephalae rhizoma*
1.5	*Gan cao*	Licorice root	*Glycyrrhizae uralensis radix*

Ma-huang and Coix Combination

Ma-huang and Coix Combination *Ma xing yi gan tang* *(Ma-hsing-i-kan-tang)*	Ephedra, Apricot Kernel, Coicis, and Licorice Decoction
Classification	*Fa biao ji:* Surface Relieving, Release Exterior Cold
Traditional Function	Dispels moisture and promotes lung qi circulation
Six Stage Relationship	*Taiyang*, water level
Pulse	Floating and rapid
Tongue	Red, thick-white coat
Abdomen	Firm
Signs and Symptoms	Body ache and fever in the evening, neuralgia, joint pain, rheumatism, rheumatoid arthritis, asthma, eczema, and warts
Contraindication	*Yang* excess

Ma-huang and Coix Combination (Composition)

4.0	*Ma huang*	Ephedra	*Epherdrae herba*
3.0	*Xing ren*	Apricot seed	*Pruni armeniacae semen*
2.0	*Gan cao*	Licorice root	*Glycyrrhizae uralensis radix*
10.0	*Yi yi ren*	Job's tears, Coxis	*Coicis lachryma-jobi*

Ma-huang and Gypsum Combination

Ma-huang and Gypsum Combination *Yue bi tang* *(Yueh-pi-tang)*	<u>Maidservant from Yue Decoction</u>
Classification	*Li shi ji:* Moisture Dispelling, Clear Heat form the Organs
Traditional Function	Dispels water and edema, soothes the lungs
Six Stage Relationship	*Tai yang,* water level
Pulse	Floating, slippery
Tongue	Red, dry-white coat
Abdomen	Soft
Signs and Symptoms	Extreme thirst, spontaneous sweating, general edema, aversion to cold, decreased urination, and cough
Contraindication	*Yang* deficiency

Ma-huang and Gypsum Combination (Composition)

6.0	*Ma huang*	Ephedra	*Epherdrae herba*
8.0	*Shi gao*	Gypsum	*Gypsum fibrosum*
3.0	*Sheng jiang*	Fresh ginger root	*Zingiberis officinalis recens rhizoma*
3.0	*Da zao*	Red date, Jujube fruit	*Ziziphi jujubae fructus*
2.0	*Gan cao*	Licorice root	*Glycyrrhizae uralensis radix*

Ma-huang and Morus Formula

Ma-huang and Morus Formula *Hua gai san* *(Hua-kai-san)*	<u>Canopy Powder</u>
Classification	*Fa biao ji:* Surface Relieving, Release Exterior Cold
Traditional Function	Suppress cough and asthma, relieves external symptoms
Six Stage Relationship	*Taiyang, qi* level
Pulse	Floating, tight
Tongue	Red, white coat
Abdomen	Firm
Signs and Symptoms	Cough and congestion in the chest due to cold wind invasion, chills and mild fever, stuffy nose, and hoarse voice
Contraindication	*Yang* deficiency

Ma-huang and Morus Formula (Composition)

4.0	*Xing ren*	Apricot seed	*Pruni armeniacae semen*
1.0	*Gan cao*	Licorice root	*Glycyrrhizae uralensis radix*
4.0	*Ma huang*	Ephedra	*Epherdrae herba*
5.0	*Fu ling*	Hoelen, Tuckahoe	*Poriae cocos sclerotium*
2.0	*Chen pi*	Tangerine peel	*Citri reticulatae pericarpium*
2.0	*Sang bai pi*	Morus bark, mulberry root bark	*Mori albae radicis cortex*
2.0	*Zi su ye*	Perilla leaf	*Perillae frutescentis folium*

Major Blue Dragon Combination

Major Blue Dragon Combination *Da qing long tang (Ta-ching-lung-tang)*	Major Blue green Dragon Decoction
Classification	*Fa biao ji:* Surface Relieving, Release Exterior Cold
Traditional Function	Clears exterior cold with internal heat
Six Stage Relationship	*Taiyang, qi* level
Pulse	Floating, tight, and rapid
Tongue	Red, thin-white or thin-yellow coat
Abdomen	Firm
Signs and Symptoms	General aching and edema, ascites, fever and chills, headaches, and thirst and anhidrosis; Delicate constitution, weak pulse and sweating
Contraindication	*Yang* excess

Major Blue Dragon Combination (Composition)

3.0	*Gui zhi*	Cinnamon twig	*Cinnamomi cassiae ramulus*
6.0	*Ma huang*	Ephedra	*Epherdrae herba*
5.0	*Xing ren*	Apricot seed	*Pruni armeniacae semen*
2.0	*Gan cao*	Licorice root	*Glycyrrhizae uralensis radix*
10.0	*Shi gao*	Gypsum	*Gypsum fibrosum*
3.0	*Sheng jiang*	Fresh ginger root	*Zingiberis officinalis recens rhizoma*
3.0	*Da zao*	Red date, Jujube fruit	*Ziziphi jujubae fructus*

Major Bupleurum Combination

Major Bupleurum Combination *Da chai hu tang* *(Ta-chai-hu-tang)*	Major Bupleurum Decoction
Classification	*Biao li shuang jie ji:* Exterior Interior Attacking, Harmonize Lesser Yang Stage Disorders
Traditional Function	Clears heat, soothes the liver, and relieves constipation
Six Stage Relationship	*Shaoyang-yangming, qi* level
Pulse	Tight and rapid, or excess deep and slow
Tongue	Red, thin-yellow coat
Abdomen	Firm
Signs and Symptoms	Gastric distress, painful hypochondriac region, alternating chills and fever, loss of appetite, constipation, and bitter taste in the mouth
Contraindication	*Yin* excess

Major Bupleurum Combination (Composition)

6.0	*Chai hu*	Bupleurum root	*Bupleuri radix*
3.0	*Huang qin*	Skullcap root, Scute	*Scutellariae baicalensis radix*
2.0	*Zhi shi*	Immature bitter orange fruit	*Citri seu ponciri immaturus fructus*
3.0	*Shao yao*	Peony	*Paeoniae radix*
1.0	*Da huang*	Rhubarb root	*Rhei radix et rhizoma*
3.0	*Ban xia (fa)*	Pinellia rhizome	*Pinelliae ternatae rhizoma*
4.0	*Sheng jiang*	Fresh ginger root	*Zingiberis officinalis recens rhizoma*
3.0	*Da zao*	Red date, Jujube fruit	*Ziziphi jujubae fructus*

Major Rhubarb Combination

Major Rhubarb Combination *Da cheng qi tang* *(Ta-cheng-chi-tang)*	Major Order the Qi Decoction
Classification	*Gong li ji:* Interior Attacking, Drain Downward
Traditional Function	Purge internal toxic heat
Six Stage Relationship	*Yangming, qi* level
Pulse	Sinking and forceful
Tongue	Red, dry-yellow to brown coat
Abdomen	Distended and full
Signs and Symptoms	Constipation, a sensation of heaviness in the body, cold sweats, extreme thirst with tidal fever, food poisoning, hypertension, mental delirium
Contraindication	Fast weak pulse with ascites, pregnancy

Major Rhubarb Combination (Composition)

2.0	*Da huang*	Rhubarb root	*Rhei radix et rhizoma*
2.0	*Mang xiao*	Mirabilite, Glauber's salt	*Mirabilitum*
5.0	*Hou po*	Magnolia bark	*Magnoliae officinalis cortex*
2.0	*Zhi shi*	Immature bitter orange fruit	*Citri seu ponciri immaturus fructus*

Major Zanthoxylum Combination

Major Zanthoxylum Combination *Da jian zhong tang* *(Ta-chien-chung-tang)*	Major Construct the Middle Decoction
Classification	*Qu han ji:* Chill Dispelling, Warm the Middle and Dispel Cold
Traditional Function	Warms the stomach and spleen, treats internal chills, abdominal pain with stagnant *qi* and water symptoms
Six Stage Relationship	*Taiyin, qi* level
Pulse	Sinking and tight
Tongue	Pale swollen, moist white coat
Abdomen	Soft, painful, and hyper-function of intestinal peristalsis
Signs and Symptoms	Intestinal constriction, intestinal flaccidity, intestinal pain due to roundworms, vomiting, and cold hands and feet
Contraindication	Overuse may cause a dry cough, edema, and vomiting

Major Zanthoxylum Combination (Composition)

5.0	*Gan jiang*	Dried ginger rhizome	*Zingiberis officinalis rhizoma*
2.0	*Chuan jiao*	Zanthoxylum, Sichuan pepper fruit	*Zanthoxyli pericarpium bungeani*
3.0	*Ren shen*	Ginseng root	*Ginseng radix*
20.0	*Jiao yi*	Maltose	*Saccharum granorum*

Melon Pedicle Formula

Melon Pedicle Formula *Gua di san* *(Kua-ti-san)*	Melon Pedicle Powder
Classification	*Cui tu ji*: Emetic, Induce Vomiting to discharge phlegm
Traditional Function	Expels excessive phlegm and stagnant food by inducing vomiting
Six Stage Relationship	*Yangming, qi* level
Pulse	Floating, slippery, full in cun position
Tongue	Red, sticky coat
Abdomen	Distended, painful
Signs and Symptoms	Food poisoning, painful distended abdomen and chest distention
Contraindication	Pregnancy, elderly or debilitated patients

Melon Pedicle Formula (Composition)

1.0	*Gua di*	Melon pedicle	*Cucumeris pedicellus*
1.0	*Chi xiao dou*	Aduki bean	*Phaseoli calcarati semen*
5.0	*Dan dou chi*	Soybean prepared	*Sojae praeparatum semen*

Minor Blue Dragon Combination

Minor Blue Dragon Combination *Xiao qing long tang* *(Hsiao-ching-lung-tang)*	Minor Blue green Dragon Decoction
Classification	*Fa biao ji:* Surface Relieving, Release Exterior Cold
Traditional Function	Relieves external symptoms, treats cough and asthma, and warms the body
Six Stage Relationship	*Taiyang, qi* level
Pulse	Floating, thin, and rapid
Tongue	Red moist, thick-white coat
Abdomen	Firm with water sounds
Signs and Symptoms	Asthmatic cough, vomiting, fever, watery and frothy sputum, decreased urination, allergies, sub cardiac edema, and general aching
Contraindication	*Yang* excess

Minor Blue Dragon Combination (Composition)

3.0	*Gui zhi*	Cinnamon twig	*Cinnamomi cassiae ramulus*
3.0	*Ma huang*	Ephedra	*Epherdrae herba*
3.0	*Wu wei zi*	Schisandra fruit	*Schisandrae chinensis fructus*
3.0	*Shao yao*	Peony	*Paeoniae radix*
3.0	*Xi xin*	Asarum, Chinese wild ginger	*Asari herba radice*
3.0	*Gan jiang*	Dried ginger rhizome	*Zingiberis officinalis rhizoma*
6.0	*Ban xia (fa)*	Pinellia rhizome	*Pinelliae ternatae rhizoma*
3.0	*Gan cao*	Licorice root	*Glycyrrhizae uralensis radix*

Minor Bupleurum Combination

Minor Bupleurum Combination *Xiao chai hu tang* *(Hsiao-chia-hu-tang)*	Minor Bupleurum Decoction
Classification	*He jie ji:* Harmonizing, Harmonize Lesser Yang-stage Disorders
Traditional Function	Treats *shaoyang* conformation, liver and gallbladder *qi* stagnation
Six Stage Relationship	*Shaoyang, qi* level
Pulse	Tight and thin or tight and rapid
Tongue	Red, thin-white coat
Abdomen	Firm with tension below the ribs and hardness beneath the heart
Signs and Symptoms	Bitter taste in the mouth, dry throat, vomiting, decreased appetite, alternating chills and fever with stomachache, abdominal pain, deafness, headache and stiffness of the neck, and difficult urination
Contraindication	*Yin* excess

Minor Bupleurum Combination (Composition)

7.0	*Chai hu*	Bupleurum root	*Bupleuri radix*
3.0	*Huang qin*	Skullcap root, Scute	*Scutellariae baicalensis radix*
5.0	*Ban xia (fa)*	Pinellia rhizome	*Pinelliae ternatae rhizoma*
4.0	*Sheng jiang*	Fresh ginger root	*Zingiberis officinalis recens rhizoma*
3.0	*Ren shen*	Ginseng root	*Ginseng radix*
3.0	*Da zao*	Red date, Jujube fruit	*Ziziphi jujubae fructus*
2.0	*Gan cao*	Licorice root	*Glycyrrhizae uralensis radix*

Minor Cinnamon and Peony Combination

Minor Cinnamon and Peony Combination *Xiao jian zhong tang* *(Hsiao-chien-chung-tang)*	Minor Construct the Middle Decoction
Classification	*Qu han ji:* Chill Dispelling, Warm the Middle and Dispel Cold
Traditional Function	Supplements qi deficiency, warms spleen and stomach, relieves pain, improves vitality in children with a delicate constitution
Six Stage Relationship	*Taiyin, qi* level
Pulse	Weak and wiry
Tongue	Pale, thin-white coat
Abdomen	Weak and painful
Signs and Symptoms	Fatigue and decreased vitality, nosebleeds, dry mouth and frequent urination, night sweats, palpitations, spasms in hands and feet, hot sensation in palms and soles, and (In children) night-crying and bed wetting
Contraindication	*Yang* excess

Minor Cinnamon and Peony Combination (Composition)

20.0	*Jiao yi*	Maltose	*Saccharum granorum*
4.0	*Da zao*	Red date, Jujube fruit	*Ziziphi jujubae fructus*
6.0	*Shao yao*	Peony	*Paeoniae radix*
2.0	*Gan cao*	Licorice root	*Glycyrrhizae uralensis radix*
4.0	*Gui zhi*	Cinnamon twig	*Cinnamomi cassiae ramulus*
4.0	*Sheng jiang*	Fresh ginger root	*Zingiberis officinalis recens rhizoma*

Minor Rhubarb Combination

Minor Rhubarb Combination *Xiao cheng qi tang* *(Hsiao-cheng-chi-tang)*	<u>Minor Order the Qi Decoction</u>
Classification	*Gong li ji:* Interior Attacking, Purge Heat Accumulation
Traditional Function	Purge *yangming* heat
Six Stage Relationship	*Yangming, qi* level
Pulse	Rapid and full, deep and slippery
Tongue	Red, sticky yellow coat
Abdomen	Distended and full
Signs and Symptoms	Tidal fever with sweating, hard stools or constipation, headaches, delirium, food poisoning, dysentery and dysuria
Contraindication	*Yin* excess, pregnancy

Minor Rhubarb Combination (Composition)

2.0	*Da huang*	Rhubarb root	*Rhei radix et rhizoma*
2.0	*Zhi shi*	Immature bitter orange fruit	*Citri seu ponciri immaturus fructus*
3.0	*Hou po*	Magnolia bark	*Magnoliae officinalis cortex*

Mume Formula

Mume Formula *Wu mei wan* *(Wu-mei-wan)*	Mume Pill
Classification	*Qu chong ji:* Anthelmintic, Expel Parasites
Traditional Function	Expels parasites, regulates qi and blood, relieves diarrhea and pain
Six Stage Relationship	*Jueyin, qi* and blood levels
Pulse	Weak
Tongue	Pale, thick white coat
Abdomen	Painful, cool due to infestation of worms
Signs and Symptoms	Abdominal pain with vomiting of ascariasis, intermittent fever and chills, anxiety and irritability, diarrhea, cold limbs, loss of appetite, a sensation of heavy pressure in the stomach, stabbing pain below the heart, accompanied by heat above the waist and cold below
Contraindication	*Yang* excess

Mume Formula (Composition)

3.0	*Wu mei*	Mume, Black plum fruit	*Pruni mume*
5.0	*Chuan jiao*	Zanthoxylum, Sichuan pepper fruit	*Zanthoxyli pericarpium bungeani*
3.0	*Xi xin*	Asarum, Chinese wild ginger	*Asari herba radice*
5.0	*Gan jiang*	Dried ginger rhizome	*Zingiberis officinalis rhizoma*
2.0	*Dang gui*	Tang kuei root	*Angelicae sinensis radix*
3.0	*Fu zi (hei)*	Prepared Sichuan aconite root	*Lateralis aconiti carmichaeli radix praeparata*
3.0	*Gui zhi*	Cinnamon twig	*Cinnamomi cassiae ramulus*
3.0	*Ren shen*	Ginseng root	*Ginseng radix*
7.0	*Huang lian*	Coptis rhizome	*Coptidis rhizoma*
3.0	*Huang bai*	Amur cork-tree bark	*Phellodendri cortex*

Ophiopogon Combination

Ophiopogon Combination *Mai men dong tang* *(Mai-men-tung-tang)*	Ophiopogonis Decoction
Classification	*Run cao ji:* Moistening, Enrich the Yin and Moisten Dryness
Traditional Function	Nourishes stomach and lung *yin* (fluids)
Six Stage Relationship	*Shaoyin* water level
Pulse	Big, weak, floating, or sinking
Tongue	Red tip, thick white or yellow coat
Abdomen	Firm with a sensation of obstruction beneath the heart
Signs and Symptoms	Facial flushing, dry cough and irritated throat, hoarseness, hypertension, dry skin, and scanty and resistant expectoration of phlegm
Contraindication	*Yang* excess

Ophiopogon Combination (Composition)

10.0	*Mai men dong*	Ophiopogon tuber, Creeping lily-turf tuber	*Ophiopogonis japonici tuber*
2.0	*Ren shen*	Ginseng root	*Ginseng radix*
5.0	*Ban xia (fa)*	Pinellia rhizome	*Pinelliae ternatae rhizoma*
2.0	*Gan cao*	Licorice root	*Glycyrrhizae uralensis radix*
3.0	*Da zao*	Red date, Jujube fruit	*Ziziphi jujubae fructus*
5.0	*Jing mi*	Rice grain	*Oryzae sativae semen*

Peony and Licorice Combination

Peony and Licorice Combination *Shao yao can cao tang* *(Shao-yao-kan-tsao-tang)*	Peony and Licorice Decoction
Classification	*He jie ji:* Harmonizing, Tonify the Blood
Traditional Function	Relieves muscular spasms and pain
Six Stage Relationship	*Jueyin,* blood level
Pulse	Weak and thin
Tongue	Red or pale
Abdomen	Weak and spasmodic
Signs and Symptoms	Muscle spasms and pain in limbs, abdomen, and back, Stiffness and pain in the shoulders, sciatica, urinary pain, and night-crying in infants
Contraindication	*Yang* excess

Peony and Licorice Combination (Composition)

6.0	*Shao yao*	Peony	*Paeoniae radix*
6.0	*Gan cao*	Licorice root	*Glycyrrhizae uralensis radix*

Persica and Rhubarb Combination

Persica and Rhubarb Combination *Tao he cheng qi tang* *(Tao-ho-cheng-chi-tang)*	Peach Pit Decoction to Order the Qi
Classification	*Li xie ji:* Blood Regulating, Invigorate the Blood and Dispel Blood Stasis
Traditional Function	Disperses stagnant blood and lumps in the lower abdomen
Six Stage Relationship	*Yangming*, blood level
Pulse	Big and full
Tongue	Red, purple, yellow coat
Abdomen	Pulsation at the abdominal artery, pain with palpable masses in lower region,
Signs and Symptoms	Constipation, painful and distended lower abdomen, headache with nervousness and over excitability, delirium, general burning sensation, palpitations, cold spasms in legs and feet, flushing up, dry mouth, abnormal menstruation and bleeding, and hypertension
Contraindication	Pregnancy

Persica and Rhubarb Combination (Composition)

5.0	*Tao ren*	Peach kernel	*Persicae semen*
4.0	*Gui zhi*	Cinnamon twig	*Cinnamomi cassiae ramulus*
1.5	*Gan cao*	Licorice root	*Glycyrrhizae uralensis radix*
3.0	*Da huang*	Rhubarb root	*Rhei radix et rhizoma*
2.0	*Mang xiao*	Mirabilite, Glauber's salt	*Mirabilitum*

Phellodendron Combination

Phellodendron Combination *Zi yin jiang huo tang* *(Tzu-yin-chiang-huo-tang)*	<u>Nourish Yin and Reduce Fire Decoction</u>
Classification	*Qing re xie huo ji:* Fire Purging
Traditional Function	Clears toxic heat and nourishes yin
Six Stage Relationship	*Shaoyang-Shaoyin*, *qi* and blood levels
Pulse	Weak, thin, and rapid
Tongue	Red, yellow-brown coat
Abdomen	Firm, hard
Signs and Symptoms	Dry cough, fever without sweating, pale, dark, dry, and withered skin, constipation and dry stools, viscid sputum, night sweats, asthma,
Contraindication	Gastrointestinal weakness and diarrhea, pallor, sweating, and cough with profuse sweating

Phellodendron Combination (Composition)

2.5	*Dang gui*	Tang kuei root	*Angelicae sinensis radix*
2.5	*Chi shao*	Red peony root	*Paeoniae rubra radix*
2.5	*Sheng di huang*	Fresh rehmannia root, Chinese foxglove root	*Rehmanniae glutinosae radix*
2.5	*Mai men dong*	Ophiopogon tuber, Creeping lily-turf tuber	*Ophiopogonis japonici tuber*
2.5	*Tian men dong*	Chinese asparagus tuber	*Asparagi cochinchinensis tuber*
1.5	*Zhi mu*	Anemarrhena root	*Anemarrhenae asphodeloidis radix*
1.5	*Huang bai*	Amur cork-tree bark	*Phellodendri cortex*
3.0	*Bai zhu*	White Atractylodes root	*Atractylodis macrocephalae rhizoma*
2.5	*Chen pi*	Tangerine peel	*Citri reticulatae pericarpium*
1.5	*Gan cao*	Licorice root	*Glycyrrhizae uralensis radix*

Picrorrhiza and Mume Combination

Picrorrhiza and Mume Combination *Lian mei an hui tang* *(Lien-mei-an-huei-tang)*	<u>Picrorrhiza and Mume Decoction to Calm</u> <u>Roundworms</u>
Classification	*Qu chong j:* Anthelmintic, Expel Parasites
Traditional Function	Expels parasites, regulates qi and blood, relieves diarrhea and pain
Six Stage Relationship	*Jueyin, qi* and blood levels
Pulse	Rapid
Tongue	Red, Thick-yellow coat
Abdomen	Parasitic abdominal pain
Signs and Symptoms	Anorexia, vomiting of ascaris, dry mouth, excess heat in liver and stomach, chills accompanied by a ruddy complexion, and somatic fever
Contraindication	*Yang* excess

Picrorrhiza and Mume Combination (Composition)

3.0	*Hu huang lian*	Amur cork-tree bark	*Phellodendri cortex*
9.0	*Lei wan*	Dragon bone	*Os draconis*
2.4	*Huang bai*	Amur cork-tree bark	*Phellodendri cortex*
2 seeds	*Wu mei*	Mume, Black plum fruit	*Pruni mume*
10 pieces	*Chuan jiao*	Zanthoxylum, Sichuan pepper fruit	*Zanthoxyli pericarpium bungeani*
2 seeds	*Bing lang*	Areca seed, Betel nut	*Arecae catechu semen*

Pinellia Combination

Pinellia Combination *Ban xiao xie xin tang* *(Pan-hsia-hsieh-hsin-tang)*	<u>Pinellia Decoction to Drain the Epigastrium</u>
Classification	*He jie ji:* Harmonizing, Harmonize Stomach and Intestines
Traditional Function	Clears damp-heat and increase the stomach and intestines
Six Stage Relationship	*Shaoyang, qi* level
Pulse	Tight, slippery, rapid
Tongue	Red, sticky-white coat
Abdomen	Distended with hardness beneath the heart
Signs and Symptoms	Gastrointestinal discomfort, borborygmus, nausea and vomiting, lack of appetite, diarrhea, and gastric acid secretion
Contraindication	*Yin* deficiency

Pinellia Combination (Composition)

1.0	*Huang lian*	Coptis rhizome	*Coptidis rhizoma*
3.0	*Huang qin*	Skullcap root, Scute	*Scutellariae baicalensis radix*
6.0	*Ban xia (fa)*	Pinellia rhizome	*Pinelliae ternatae rhizoma*
3.0	*Gan jiang*	Dried ginger rhizome	*Zingiberis officinalis rhizoma*
3.0	*Ren shen*	Ginseng root	*Ginseng radix*
3.0	*Gan cao*	Licorice root	*Glycyrrhizae uralensis radix*
3.0	*Da zao*	Red date, Jujube fruit	*Ziziphi jujubae fructus*

Pinellia and Ginger Combination

Pinellia and Ginger Combination *Sheng jiang xie xin tang* *(Sheng-chiang-hsieh-hsin-tang)*	<u>Fresh Ginger Decoction to Drain the Epigastrium</u>
Classification	*He jie ji:* Harmonizing, Harmonize the Stomach and Intestines
Traditional Function	Clears damp heat and qi stagnation the stomach and intestines, and promotes digestion
Six Stage Relationship	*Shaoyang, qi* level
Pulse	Full and slippery
Tongue	Red, thick-white or yellow coat
Abdomen	Distended with sucussion sounds
Signs and Symptoms	Gastrointestinal disorders, borborygmus and diarrhea, sour stomach
Contraindication	*Yin* deficiency

Pinellia and Ginger Combination (Composition)

1.0	*Huang lian*	Coptis rhizome	*Coptidis rhizoma*
2.5	*Huang qin*	Skullcap root, Scute	*Scutellariae baicalensis radix*
5.0	*Ban xia (fa)*	Pinellia rhizome	*Pinelliae ternatae rhizoma*
1.5	*Gan jiang*	Dried ginger rhizome	*Zingiberis officinalis rhizoma*
2.5	*Ren shen*	Ginseng root	*Ginseng radix*
2.5	*Gan cao*	Licorice root	*Glycyrrhizae uralensis radix*
2.5	*Da zao*	Red date, Jujube fruit	*Ziziphi jujubae fructus*
2.0	*Sheng jiang*	Fresh ginger root	*Zingiberis officinalis recens rhizoma*

Pinellia and Licorice Combination

Pinellia and Licorice Combination *Gan cao xie xin tang* *(Kan-tsao-hsieh-hsin-tang)*	Licorice Decoction to Drain the Epigastrium
Classification	*He jie ji:* Harmonizing, Harmonizing the Stomach and Intestines
Traditional Function	Treats stress related gastrointestinal complaints with symptoms of distention beneath the heart
Six Stage Relationship	*Shaoyang, qi* level
Pulse	Full and tight
Tongue	Red, white or thin-yellow coat
Abdomen	Borborygmus with obstruction and hardening below the heart
Signs and Symptoms	Loss of appetite, frequent diarrhea, mental instability, nervous exhaustion and insomnia, and retching
Contraindication	*Yang* excess

Pinellia and Licorice Combination (Composition)

1.0	*Huang lian*	Coptis rhizome	*Coptidis rhizoma*
2.5	*Huang qin*	Skullcap root, Scute	*Scutellariae baicalensis radix*
5.0	*Ban xia (fa)*	Pinellia rhizome	*Pinelliae ternatae rhizoma*
2.5	*Gan jiang*	Dried ginger rhizome	*Zingiberis officinalis rhizoma*
2.5	*Ren shen*	Ginseng root	*Ginseng radix*
3.5	*Gan cao*	Licorice root	*Glycyrrhizae uralensis radix*
2.5	*Da zao*	Red date, Jujube fruit	*Ziziphi jujubae fructus*

Polyporus Combination

Polyporus Combination *Zhu ling tang* *(Chu-ling-tang)*	Polyporus Decoction
Classification	*Li shi ji:* Moisture Dispelling, Promote Urination and Leech Out Dampness
Traditional Function	Clears damp-heat in the lower *jiao*, nourishes the *yin*
Six Stage Relationship	*Yangming,* water level
Pulse	Floating and rapid
Tongue	Red, sticky yellow coat
Abdomen	Distended and full in lower region
Signs and Symptoms	Hematuria, painful and difficult urination, fever, insomnia, extreme thirst and chest discomfort, diarrhea, and edema below the waist
Contraindication	*Yang* deficiency

Polyporus Combination (Composition)

3.0	*Zhu ling*	Polyporus	*Polypori umbellati sclerotium*
3.0	*Fu ling*	Hoelen, Tuckahoe	*Poriae cocos sclerotium*
3.0	*Ze xie*	Water plantain rhizome	*Alismatis orientalis rhizoma*
3.0	*Hua shi*	Talc, Soapstone	*Talcum*
3.0	*E jiao*	Donkey hide gelatin, Ass skin glue	*Asini cori gelatinum*

Pueraria Combination

Pueraria Combination *Ge gen tang* *(Ko-ken-tang)*	Kudzu Decoction
Classification	*Fa biao ji:* Surface Relieving, Release Exterior with Head and Neck Symptoms
Traditional Function	Treats external wind-cold symptoms and harmonizes *ying qi* and *wei qi*
Six Stage Relationship	*Taiyang-shaoyang, qi* level
Pulse	Floating, tight, and rapid
Tongue	Red, thin white coat
Abdomen	Firm
Signs and Symptoms	Headache, stiffness and pain in neck and upper back, fever and chills without sweating, diarrhea, painful urination, and general aching and muscle spasms
Contraindication	*Yin* deficiency

Pueraria Combination (Composition)

8.0	*Ge gen*	Kudzu root	*Puerariae radix*
3.0	*Shao yao*	Peony	*Paeoniae radix*
3.0	*Gui zhi*	Cinnamon twig	*Cinnamomi cassiae ramulus*
4.0	*Ma huang*	Ephedra	*Epherdrae herba*
1.0	*Gan jiang*	Dried ginger rhizome	*Zingiberis officinalis rhizoma*
4.0	*Da zao*	Red date, Jujube fruit	*Ziziphi jujubae fructus*
2.0	*Gan cao*	Licorice root	*Glycyrrhizae uralensis radix*

Pueraria, Coptis, and Scute Combination

Pueraria, Coptis, and Scute Combination *Ge gen huang lian huang qin tang* *(Ko-ken-huang-lien-huang-chin-tang)*	Kudzu, Coptis, and Scutellaria Decoction
Classification	*Biao li shuang jie ji:* Exterior Interior Attacking, Release Exterior Interior Excess
Traditional Function	Clears internal heat caused by wind-cold invasion
Six Stage Relationship	*Taiyang-shaoyang, qi* level
Pulse	Sinking and tight
Tongue	Red, thin white coat
Abdomen	Painful, obstruction beneath the heart, tenesmus in lower abdomen
Signs and Symptoms	Fever, feverish sensation in the chest, perspiration, stiffness and spasms in neck and upper back, palpitations, mental instability, diarrhea and stomachache
Contraindication	*Yin* excess

Pueraria, Coptis, and Scute Combination (Composition)

6.0	*Ge gen*	Kudzu root	*Puerariae radix*
2.0	*Gan cao*	Licorice root	*Glycyrrhizae uralensis radix*
3.0	*Huang lian*	Coptis rhizome	*Coptidis rhizoma*
3.0	*Huang qin*	Skullcap root, Scute	*Scutellariae baicalensis radix*

Rhubarb and Aconite Combination

Rhubarb and Aconite Combination *Da huang fu zi tang* *(Ta-huang-fu-tzu-tang)*	Rhubarb and Prepared Aconite Decoction
Classification	*Gong li ji:* Interior Attacking, Moisten the Intestines and Unblock the Bowels
Traditional Function	Purge stagnation in the middle and lower *jiaos* and dispels cold
Six Stage Relationship	*Yangming-Jueyin, qi* level
Pulse	Sinking and tight
Tongue	Pale, white coat
Abdomen	Soft with mild tension, unilateral pain right hypochondriac region, and spasms beside and below the umbilicus
Signs and Symptoms	Constipation, pain and cold below the waist, pain in the armpits, waist, and legs, gastric and intestinal spasms, pain caused by kidney stones or gallstones, sciatica, and inercostal neuralgia
Contraindication	*Yang* excess, pregnancy

Rhubarb and Aconite Combination (Composition)

1.0	*Da huang*	Rhubarb root	*Rhei radix et rhizoma*
0.5-1.0	*Fu zi (hei)*	Prepared Sichuan aconite root	*Lateralis aconiti carmichaeli radix praeparata*
2.0	*Xi xin*	Asarum, Chinese wild ginger	*Asari herba radice*

Rhubarb, Ginger, and Croton Combination

Rhubarb, Ginger, and Croton Combination *San wu bei ji wan* *(San-wu-pei-chi-wan)*	<u>Rhubarb, Ginger, and Croton Decoction</u>
Classification	*Gong li ji:* Interior Attacking
Traditional Function	Purge stagnation due to cold
Six Stage Relationship	*Yangming, qi* level
Pulse	Tight
Tongue	Thick-white coat
Abdomen	Painful and distended
Signs and Symptoms	Abdominal distention and pain due to cold or ingestion of cold food, rapid breathing and severe pain
Contraindication	Do not take in large amounts as *Ba* dou is a poisonous herb. It is safe in small doses when correctly processed, pregnancy.

Rhubarb, Ginger, and Croton Combination (Composition)

1.0	*Da huang*	Rhubarb root	*Rhei radix et rhizoma*
1.0	*Ba dou*	Croton seed	*Croton tiglii semen*
1.0	*Gan jiang*	Dried ginger rhizome	*Zingiberis officinalis rhizoma*

Rhubarb and Kan-sui Combination

Rhubarb and Kan-sui Combination *Da xian xiong tang* *(Ta-hsien-hsiung-tang)*	<u>Major Sinking Into the Chest Decoction</u>
Classification	*Gong li ji:* Interior Attacking
Traditional Function	Purge internal damp heat
Six Stage Relationship	*Yangming-Shaoyin,* water level
Pulse	Slippery and rapid
Tongue	Red, sticky white-yellow coat
Abdomen	Sub cardiac distention and pain
Signs and Symptoms	Severe chest pain with sub cardiac distention and constipation, dry mouth, thirst, shortness of breath, restlessness evening tidal fever, pulmonary edema, and intercostal neuralgia
Contraindication	Weak persons with a delicate constitution, pregnancy

Rhubarb and Kan-sui Combination (Composition)

9.0	*Da huang*	Rhubarb root	*Rhei radix et rhizoma*
1.5	*Mang xiao*	Mirabilite, Glauber's salt	*Mirabilitum*
1.5	*Gan sui*	Kansui spurge root	*Euphorbiae kansui radix*

Rhubarb and Leech Combination

Rhubarb and Leech Combination *Di dang tang* *(Ti-tang-tang)*	<u>Resistance Decoction</u>
Classification	*Li xie ji:* Blood Regulating, Invigorate the Blood and Dispel Blood Stasis
Traditional Function	Activates, purge, and regulates stagnant blood
Six Stage Relationship	*Yangming,* blood level
Pulse	Thin, firm
Tongue	Dark-red, white or yellow coat
Abdomen	Distended and painful, hard masses in the lower abdomen
Signs and Symptoms	Constipation with swelling and pain in the lower abdomen, resistance and pain when pressing the abdomen, dark stools, amenorrhea, amnesia and anxiety, and external injuries
Contraindication	*Yang* excess, pregnancy

Rhubarb and Leech Combination (Composition)

1.0	*Shui zhi*	Leech	*Hirudo seu whitmania*
1.0	*Meng chong*	Gadfly	*Tabani Bivittati*
1.0	*Tao ren*	Peach kernel	*Persicae semen*
3.0	*Da huang*	Rhubarb root	*Rhei radix et rhizoma*

Rhubarb and Mirabilitum Combination

Rhubarb and Mirabilitum Combination *Tiao wei cheng qi tang* *(Tiao-wei-cheng-chi-tang)*	Regulate the Stomach and Order the Qi Decoction
Classification	*Gong li ji:* Interior Attacking, Purge Heat Accumulation
Traditional Function	Purge stagnant heat, lubricates bowels
Six Stage Relationship	*Yangming, qi* level
Pulse	Sinking tight, excessive
Tongue	Red and dry
Abdomen	Distended and painful to pressure
Signs and Symptoms	Constipation and dry stools, upset stomach, dry mouth and tongue, constipation in the elderly, aversion to heat, acute gastrointeritis, and food poisoning
Contraindication	*Yin* excess, pregnancy

Rhubarb and Mirabilitum Combination (Composition)

2.5	*Da huang*	Rhubarb root	*Rhei radix et rhizoma*
1.0	*Mang xiao*	Mirabilite, Glauber's salt	*Mirabilitum*
1.0	*Gan cao*	Licorice root	*Glycyrrhizae uralensis radix*

Rhubarb and Moutan Combination

Rhubarb and Moutan Combination *Da huang mu dan pi tang (Ta-huang-mu-tan-pi-tang)*	Rhubarb and Moutan Decoction
Classification	*Yong yang ji:* Carbuncle Dermatosis, Purge Heat Accumulation
Traditional Function	Clears internal heat, disperses hard masses and blood stagnation, reduces carbuncles
Six Stage Relationship	*Yangming,* blood level
Pulse	Tight and slow
Tongue	Red, sticky yellow
Abdomen	Swollen and painful, fever in lower abdomen, tumor or hard lump in lower right quadrant
Signs and Symptoms	Frequent fever with constipation, spontaneous sweating, fever with suppuration, tumors or lumps in lower abdomen, acute appendicitis, hemorrhoids and rectal prolapse
Contraindication	Pregnancy

Rhubarb and Moutan Combination (Composition)

2.0	*Da huang*	Rhubarb root	*Rhei radix et rhizoma*
4.0	*Mang xiao*	Mirabilite, Glauber's salt	*Mirabilitum*
4.0	*Mu dan pi*	Tree peony root-bark	*Moutan radicis cortex*
4.0	*Tao ren*	Peach kernel	*Persicae semen*
6.0	*Dong gua zi*	Benincasa	*Benincasae semen*

Schizonepeta and Siler Combination

Schizonepeta and Siler Combination *Jing fang bai du san* *(Ching-fang-pai-tu-san)*	Schizonepeta and Ledebouriella Powder to Overcome Pathogenic Influences
Classification	*Yong yang ji:* Carbuncle Dermatosis, Release Exterior Disorders with Interior Deficiency
Traditional Function	Reduces inflammation and swelling by dispersing wind and cold
Six Stage Relationship	*Taiyang,* blood level
Pulse	Floating and tight
Tongue	Red, thin-white coat
Abdomen	Firm
Signs and Symptoms	Fever and chills, headache, initial stage of suppuration, boils, carbuncles, mastitis, eczema, dermatitis, muscle spasms, and pustules
Contraindication	*Yin* excess

Schizonepeta and Siler Combination (Composition)

1.5	*Chai hu*	Bupleurum root	*Bupleuri radix*
1.5	*Qian hu*	Hogfennel root, Peucedanum	*Peucedani radix*
1.5	*Bo he*	Field Mint	*Menthae herba*
1.0	*Gan jiang*	Dried ginger rhizome	*Zingiberis officinalis rhizoma*
1.5	*Jing jie*	Schizonepeta stem or bud	*Schizonepetae tenuifoliae herba seu flos*
1.5	*Fang feng*	Siler root	*Ledebouriellae divaricatae radix*
1.5	*Qiang huo*	Notopterygium rhizome and root	*Notopterygii rhizoma et radix*
1.5	*Du huo*	Angelica root pubescent	*Angelicae pubescentis radix*
1.5	*Lian jiao*	Ephedra	*Epherdrae herba*
1.5	*Jin yin hua*	Honeysuckle Flower	*Lonicerae japonicae flos*
1.5	*Jie geng (ku)*	Balloon flower root, Platycodon	*Platycodi grandiflori radix*
1.5	*Chuan xiong*	Szechuan lovage root	*Ligustici chuanxiong radix*
1.5	*Zhi ke*	Bitter orange fruit	*Citri aurantii fructus*
1.0	*Gan cao*	Licorice root	*Glycyrrhizae uralensis radix*

Scute and Licorice Combination

Scute and Licorice Combination *Huang qin tang* *(Huang-chin-tang)*	Scutellaria Decoction
Classification	*He jie ji:* Harmonizing, Clear Damp Heat
Traditional Function	Clears damp-heat and relieves spasms
Six Stage Relationship	*Taiyang-yangming,* water level
Pulse	Rapid
Tongue	Red, yellow coat
Abdomen	Spasms in the right rectus abdominis muscle, a sensation of obstruction beneath the heart, and pain around the umbilical region
Signs and Symptoms	Hot diarrhea, dysentery, mucous like or tarry stools, fever, headache, extreme thirst, vomiting, and spasmodic contraction of the anal sphincter
Contraindication	*Yin* excess

Scute and Licorice Combination (Composition)

4.0	*Huang qin*	Skullcap root, Scute	*Scutellariae baicalensis radix*
3.0	*Shao yao*	Peony	*Paeoniae radix*
3.0	*Gan cao*	Licorice root	*Glycyrrhizae uralensis radix*
4.0	*Da zao*	Red date, Jujube fruit	*Ziziphi jujubae fructus*

Siler and Platycodon Formula

Siler and Platycodon Formula *Fang feng tong sheng san* *(Fang-feng-tung-sheng-san)*	<u>Ledebouriella Powder that Sagely Unblocks</u>
Classification	*Biao li shuang jie ji:* Exterior-Interior Attacking, Release Exterior-Interior Excess
Traditional Function	Promotes sweating and purge internal heat
Six Stage Relationship	*Taiyang-yangming, qi* level
Pulse	Rapid and full, wiry
Tongue	Red, dark red, dry yellow coat
Abdomen	Tight fullness
Signs and Symptoms	Obese constitution, hypertension, habitual constipation, stiffness in shoulders, fatigue, heaviness in the head, numbness in hands and feet, and yellow-white skin with facial flushing
Contraindication	*Yin* deficient

Siler and Platycodon Formula (Composition)

1.5	*Da huang*	Rhubarb root	*Rhei radix et rhizoma*
1.5	*Mang xiao*	Mirabilite, Glauber's salt	*Mirabilitum*
2.0	*Gan cao*	Licorice root	*Glycyrrhizae uralensis radix*
1.2	*Fang feng*	Siler root	*Ledebouriellae divaricatae radix*
1.2	*Ma huang*	Ephedra	*Epherdrae herba*
1.2	*Sheng jiang*	Fresh ginger root	*Zingiberis officinalis recens rhizoma*
2.0	*Jie geng (ku)*	Balloon flower root, Platycodon	*Platycodi grandiflori radix*
1.2	*Zhi zi*	Gardenia fruit	*Gardenia jasminoidis fructus*
1.2	*Lian jiao*	Ephedra	*Epherdrae herba*
1.2	*Jing jie*	Schizonepeta stem or bud	*Schizonepetae tenuifoliae herba seu flos*
1.2	*Bo he*	Field Mint	*Menthae herba*
2.0	*Bai zhu*	White Atractylodes root	*Atractylodis macrocephalae rhizoma*
3.0	*Hua shi*	Talc, Soapstone	*Talcum*

2.0	*Huang qin*	Skullcap root, Scute	*Scutellariae baicalensis radix*
2.0	*Shi gao*	Gypsum	*Gypsum fibrosum*
1.2	*Dang gui*	Tang kuei root	*Angelicae sinensis radix*
1.2	*Shao yao*	Peony	*Paeoniae radix*
1.2	*Chuan xiong*	Szechuan lovage root	*Ligustici chuanxiong radix*

Six Major Herb Combination

Six Major Herb Combination *Liu jun zi tang* *(Liu-chun-tzu-tang)*	Six-Gentleman Decoction
Classification	*Bu yi ji:* Tonic and Replenishing, Tonify the *Qi*
Traditional Function	Increase spleen *qi*
Six Stage Relationship	*Taiyin, qi* and water levels
Pulse	Weak, mildly slippery
Tongue	Pale, flabby, thin-white coat
Abdomen	Soft and weak with sucussion sounds
Signs and Symptoms	Fatigue and general weakness, chronic gastro-intestinal disorders, poor appetite, distention below the heart, weight loss, and anemia
Contraindication	*Yang* excess

Six Major Herb Combination (Composition)

4.0	*Ren shen*	Ginseng root	*Ginseng radix*
4.0	*Bai zhu*	White Atractylodes root	*Atractylodis macrocephalae rhizoma*
4.0	*Fu ling*	Hoelen, Tuckahoe	*Poriae cocos sclerotium*
1.0	*Gan cao*	Licorice root	*Glycyrrhizae uralensis radix*
2.0	*Chen pi*	Tangerine peel	*Citri reticulatae pericarpium*
4.0	*Ban xia (fa)*	Pinellia rhizome	*Pinelliae ternatae rhizoma*
2.0	*Sheng jiang*	Fresh ginger root	*Zingiberis officinalis recens rhizoma*
2.0	*Da zao*	Red date, Jujube fruit	*Ziziphi jujubae fructus*

Tang kuei and Arctium

Tang kuei and Arctium Formula *Xiao feng san* *(Hsiao feng san)*	Eliminate Wind Powder from True Lineage
Classification	*Qu feng ji:* Wind Dispelling, Release Wind from the Skin and Channels
Traditional Function	Dispels wind and eliminates itching, cools blood
Six Stage Relationship	*Yangming-Taiyin,* blood level
Pulse	Floating and rapid
Tongue	Red tip, white or yellow coat
Abdomen	Firm
Signs and Symptoms	Itching weeping rash due to wind-heat invasion, purpura, recalcitrant eczema, skin diseases aggravated by hot-damp weather, chronic urticaria, and prickly heat sensation
Contraindication	*Yang* excess, pregnancy

Tang kuei and Arctium Formula (Composition)

3.0	*Dang gui*	Tang kuei root	*Angelicae sinensis radix*
3.0	*Sheng di huang*	Fresh rehmannia root, Chinese foxglove root	*Rehmanniae glutinosae radix*
1.5	*Hu ma ren*	Sesame	*Sesami radix*
1.0	*Ku shen*	Sophora Root, Bitter ginseng root	*Sophorae flavescentis radix*
1.5	*Zhi mu*	Anemarrhena root	*Anemarrhenae asphodeloidis radix*
3.0	*Shi gao*	Gypsum	*Gypsum fibrosum*
2.0	*Niu bang zi*	Burdock fruit	*Arctii lappae fructus*
1.0	*Chan tui*	Red peony root	*Paeoniae rubra radix*
1.0	*Jing jie*	Schizonepeta stem or bud	*Schizonepetae tenuifoliae herba seu flos*
2.0	*Fang feng*	Siler root	*Ledebouriellae divaricatae radix*
2.0	*Mu tong*	Akebia stem	*Mutong caulis*
2.0	*Cang zhu*	Atractylodes rhizome	*Atractylodis rizoma*
1.0	*Gan cao*	Licorice root	*Glycyrrhizae uralensis radix*

Tang-kuei and Gardenia Combination

Tang-kuei and Gardenia Combination *Wen qing yin* (*Wen-ching-yin*)	Warm and Clearing Decoction
Classification	*Li xie ji:* Blood Regulating, Tonify the Blood
Traditional Function	Activates, cools, and disperses stagnant blood
Six Stage Relationship	*Taiyin*, blood level
Pulse	Rapid, tight, or slippery
Tongue	Red tip, yellow coat
Abdomen	Distension in the upper abdomen
Signs and Symptoms	Brown-yellow, or brownish dry skin, mouth and tongue ulcers, ulcers on the external genitals, uterine bleeding, emotional instability, and hypertension
Contraindication	*Yang* excess, pregnancy

Tang-kuei and Gardenia Combination (Composition)

4.0	*Dang gui*	Tang kuei root	*Angelicae sinensis radix*
4.0	*Sheng di huang*	Fresh rehmannia root, Chinese foxglove root	*Rehmanniae glutinosae radix*
3.0	*Shao yao*	Peony	*Paeoniae radix*
3.0	*Chuan xiong*	Szechuan lovage root	*Ligustici chuanxiong radix*
1.5	*Huang lian*	Coptis rhizome	*Coptidis rhizoma*
3.0	*Huang qin*	Skullcap root, Scute	*Scutellariae baicalensis radix*
1.5	*Huang bai*	Amur cork-tree bark	*Phellodendri cortex*
2.0	*Zhi zi*	Gardenia fruit	*Gardenia jasminoidis fructus*

Tang-kuei and Ginseng Eight Combination

Tang-kuei and Ginseng Eight Combination *Ba zheng tang* *(Pa-chen-tang)*	Eight-treasure Decoction
Classification	*Bu yi ji:* Tonic and Replenishing, Tonify *Qi* and Blood
Traditional Function	Increase *qi* and blood deficiency
Six Stage Relationship	*Taiyin*, blood level
Pulse	Weak and thin
Tongue	Pale and shaky
Abdomen	Distended lower abdomen and painful lower back
Signs and Symptoms	Anemia, dizziness, fatigue and debility, poor digestion, general weakness during convalescence, lower abdominal distention, irregular menstruation, and liver and spleen blood deficiency
Contraindication	*Yang* excess

Tang-kuei and Ginseng Eight Combination (Composition)

3.0	*Dang gui*	Tang kuei root	*Angelicae sinensis radix*
3.0	*Shu di huang*	Wine cooked rehmannia, Foxglove	*Rehmanniae glutinosae conquitae radix*
3.0	*Shao yao*	Peony	*Paeoniae radix*
3.0	*Chuan xiong*	Szechuan lovage root	*Ligustici chuanxiong radix*
3.0	*Ren shen*	Ginseng root	*Ginseng radix*
3.0	*Bai zhu*	White Atractylodes root	*Atractylodis macrocephalae rhizoma*
3.0	*Fu ling*	Hoelen, Tuckahoe	*Poriae cocos sclerotium*
1.5	*Gan cao*	Licorice root	*Glycyrrhizae uralensis radix*
1.5	*Da zao*	Red date, Jujube fruit	*Ziziphi jujubae fructus*
1.5	*Sheng jiang*	Fresh ginger root	*Zingiberis officinalis recens rhizoma*

Tang-kuei and Jujube Combination

Tang-kuei and Jujube Combination *Dang gui si ni tang* *(Tang-kuei-szu-ni-tang)*	<u>Tang kuei Decoction for Frigid Extremities</u>
Classification	*Qu han ji:* Chill Dispelling, Warm the Channels and Disperse Cold
Traditional Function	Warms the body, moves and nourishes the blood
Six Stage Relationship	*Taiyin Jueyin,* blood level
Pulse	Weak, deep and thin
Tongue	Pale, white coat
Abdomen	Tension upon light palpation but soft and tender with deep pressure, weak
Signs and Symptoms	Cold (purple) hands and feet, cold sweats, weak and spasmodic abdomen, diarrhea, annoying fullness in the chest, cough with clear sputum, frostbite, and cold limbs as a result of over use of diaphoretics
Contraindication	*Yang* excess

Tang-kuei and Jujube Combination (Composition)

3.0	*Dang gui*	Tang kuei root	*Angelicae sinensis radix*
3.0	*Gui zhi*	Cinnamon twig	*Cinnamomi cassiae ramulus*
2.0	*Xi xin*	Asarum, Chinese wild ginger	*Asari herba radice*
3.0	*Mu tong*	Akebia stem	*Mutong caulis*
5.0	*Da zao*	Red date, Jujube fruit	*Ziziphi jujubae fructus*
2.0	*Gan cao*	Licorice root	*Glycyrrhizae uralensis radix*
3.0	*Shao yao*	Peony	*Paeoniae radix*

Tang-kuei and Jujube Combination

Trichosanthes and Chih-shih Combination *Gua lou zhi shi tang* *(Kua-lou-chih-shih-tang)*	Trichosanthes Fruit and Immature Bitter Orange Decoction
Classification	*Qu tan ji:* Expectorant, Clear Heat and Transform Phlegm
Traditional Function	Regulates qi, clears heat in the upper jiao, and dissolves phlegm
Six Stage Relationship	*Taiyang-Shaoyin*, water level
Pulse	Rapid and slippery
Tongue	Red, sticky white coat
Abdomen	Firm, and painful
Signs and Symptoms	Viscous, dry and yellow phlegm, chest pain and difficult breathing, fullness and discomfort in the chest, angina pectorus, speech impairment, intercostal neuralgia, hypertension, red urine, and smoker's cough
Contraindication	*Yin* excess

Trichosanthes and Chih-shih Combination (Composition)

1.0	*Zhi zi*	Gardenia fruit	*Gardenia jasminoidis fructus*
2.0	*Huang qin*	Skullcap root, Scute	*Scutellariae baicalensis radix*
3.0	*Dang gui*	Tang kuei root	*Angelicae sinensis radix*
1.0	*Gan cao*	Licorice root	*Glycyrrhizae uralensis radix*
2.0	*Gua lou ren*	Snakegourd seed	*Trichosanthis semen*
3.0	*Bei mu*	Fritillaria	*Fritillariae bulbus*
1.0	*Zhu li*	Dried bamboo sap	*Bambusae succus*
2.0	*Sheng jiang*	Fresh ginger root	*Zingiberis officinalis recens rhizoma*
1.0	*Zhi shi*	Immature bitter orange fruit	*Citri seu ponciri immaturus fructus*
2.0	*Chen pi*	Tangerine peel	*Citri reticulatae pericarpium*
1.0	*Suo sha*	Cardamon	*Amoni semen*
1.0	*Mu xiang*	Saussurea	*Natrium sulphuricum*
3.0	*Fu ling*	Hoelen, Tuckahoe	*Poriae cocos sclerotium*
2.0	*Jie geng (ku)*	Balloon flower root, Platycodon	*Platycodi grandiflori radix*

Trichosanthes, Barkeri, and Pinellia Combination

Trichosanthes, Barkeri, and Pinellia Combination *Gua lou xie bai ban xia tang* *(Kua-lou-hsieh-pai-pan-hsia-tang)*	<u>Immature Bitter Orange, Trichosanthes Fruit, and Cinnamon Twig Decoction</u>
Classification	*Li qi ji: Qi* Regulating, Promote the Movement of *Qi*
Traditional Function	Disperses stagnation and phlegm in the upper *jiao* with *yang* deficiency
Six Stage Relationship	*Shaoyin, qi* and water levels
Pulse	Irregular, slippery
Tongue	Pale, light purple, wet, white coat
Abdomen	Obstruction and hardening below the heart, lower abdomen weak
Signs and Symptoms	Pain in the sternum and around the heart, labored breathing, heart pain that radiates into the back, cough, and angina pectorus
Contraindication	*Yin* deficiency

Trichosanthes, Barkeri, and Pinellia Combination (Composition)

3.0	*Gua lou gen*	Tricosanthes root	*Trichosanthis radix*
4.5	*Xie bai*	Bakeri, Chinese chive bulb	*Allii bulbus macrostemi*
3.0	*Ban xia (fa)*	Pinellia rhizome	*Pinelliae ternatae rhizoma*

Vitality Combination

Vitality Combination *Zhen wu tang* *(Chen-wu-tang)*	<u>True Warrior Decoction</u>
Classification	*Qu han ji:* Chill Dispelling, Clear Damp Heat
Traditional Function	Increase yang, warms the interior, promotes water metabolism
Six Stage Relationship	*Taiyin-Shaoyin,* qi and water levels
Pulse	Deep and minute, floating and weak
Tongue	Pale, thin-white coat
Abdomen	Soft, weak, painful, and distended
Signs and Symptoms	Fatigue, aching and heaviness of the limbs, watery diarrhea, valvular disease, palpitations, edema, decreased and clear urine, and trembling of the body
Contraindication	*Yang* excess

Vitality Combination (Composition)

0.5-1.0	*Fu zi (hei)*	Prepared Sichuan aconite root	*Lateralis aconiti carmichaeli radix praeparata*
3.0	*Sheng jiang*	Fresh ginger root	*Zingiberis officinalis recens rhizoma*
3.0	*Bai zhu*	White Atractylodes root	*Atractylodis macrocephalae rhizoma*
5.0	*Fu ling*	Hoelen, Tuckahoe	*Poriae cocos sclerotium*
3.0	*Shao yao*	Peony	*Paeoniae radix*

Zizyphus Combination

Zizyphus Combination *Suan zao ren tang* *(Suan-Tsao-jen-Tang)*	Sour Jujube Decoction
Classification	*Zhen jing ji:* Sedative, Nourish the Heart and Calm the Spirit
Traditional Function	Calms irritability in the heart and pacifies the *shen*
Six Stage Relationship	*Shaoyin, qi* level
Pulse	Weak, irregular
Tongue	Red tip, white coat
Abdomen	Weak and soft
Signs and Symptoms	Cardiac hyper function, palpitations, insomnia, discomfort in the chest, night sweats, fatigue, vertigo, and absent-mindedness
Contraindication	*Yang* excess

Zizyphus Combination (Composition)

10.0	*Suan zao ren*	Zizyphus seed, Sour jujube	*Zizyphi spinosae semen*
5.0	*Fu ling*	Hoelen, Tuckahoe	*Poriae cocos sclerotium*
3.0	*Chuan xiong*	Szechuan lovage root	*Ligustici chuanxiong radix*
1.0	*Gan cao*	Licorice root	*Glycyrrhizae uralensis radix*
3.0	*Zhi mu*	Anemarrhena root	*Anemarrhenae asphodeloidis radix*

Chapter Eleven

Individual Herb Lists

Overview

The main emphasis in this section is on a cross reference for the most commonly used individual herbs. The herbs can be found by their *Pin Yin* name, Pharmaceutical name, and Common name. The last part of this section (Classification and Function List) is a quick reference for only the herbs used in this book. There are one hundred and fifteen individual herbs used in this book listed by their *Pin Yin* name.

1. *Pin Yin* List
2. Pharmaceutical List
3. Common Name List
4. Classification and Function List

Pinyin (Herb List)

Pin Yin	Pharmaceutical	Common Name
Ai ye	Artemisiae argyi folium	Mugwort leaf
An xi xiang	Benzoinum	Styrax benzoin processed resin
Ba dou	Croton tiglii semen	Croton seed
Ba ji tian	Morindae officinalis radix	Morinda root
Ba qia	Smilacis china rizoma	Smilax rhizome
Bai dou kou	Amomi cardamomi fructus	Cardamon fruit
Bai dou kou	Amomi kravanh fructus	Cardamon white
Bai guo	Ginkgo bilobae semen	Ginkgo seed
Bai he	Lilii bulbus	Lily bulb
Bai hua she she cao	Oldenlandiae diffusae herba	Oldenlandia
Bai ji li	Tribuli terrestris fructus	Caltrop fruit
Bai jiang cao	Patriniae heterophyllae herba	Thiaspi, Patrinia
Bai mao gen	Imperatae cylindricae rhizoma	Imperata rhizome
Bai shao	Paeoniae lactiflorae radix	White Peony root
Bai tou weng	Pulsatillae chinensis radix	Pulsatilla root
Bai xian pi	Dictamni dasycarpi radicis cortex	Dittany root bark
Bai zhi	Angelicae dahurica radix	Angelica root
Bai zhu	Atractylodis macrocephalae rhizoma	White Atractylodes root
Bai zi ren	Biotae orientalis semen	Biota seed
Ban lan gen	Isatidis seu baphicacanthi radix	Woad root
Ban xia	Pinellia tuber	Pinellia
Ban xia (fa)	Pinelliae ternatae rhizoma	Pinellia rhizome
Ban xia (sheng)	Pinelliae tematae rhizome	Prepared Pinellia rhizome
Bei mu	Fritillariae bulbus	Fritillaria
Bei xie	Dioscorae hypoglaucae rhizome	Tokoro, Yam rhizome
Bing lang	Arecae catechu semen	Areca seed, Betel nut
Bo he	Menthae herba	Field Mint
Bo he	Menthae haplocalycis herba	Mint
Bo he	Mentha herba	Mentha
Bu gu zhi	Psoraleae corylifoliae fructus	Scuffy Pea
Can sha	Bombycis mori excrementum	Silkworm feces
Cang er zi	Xanthii fructus	Xanthium, Cocklebur fruit
Cang zhu	Atractylodis rizoma	Atractylodes rhizome

Pin Yin	Pharmaceutical	Common Name
Cang zhu	*Atractylodis rizoma*	Atractylodes rhizome (red)
Ce bai ye	*Biotae orientalis cacumen*	Biota leaf
Cha ye	*Camelliae folium*	Tea
Chai hu	*Bupleuri radix*	Bupleurum root
Che qian zi	*Plantaginis semen*	Plantago seed
Chen pi	*Citri reticulatae pericarpium*	Tangerine peel
Chi shao	*Paeoniae rubra radix*	Red peony root
Chi xiao dou	*Phaseoli calcarati semen*	Aduki bean
Chu shi zi	*Broussonetie fructus*	Broussonetia fruit
Chuan bei mu	*Fritillariae cirrhosae bulbus*	Fritillaria bulb
Chuan jiao	*Zanthoxyli pericarpium bungeani*	Zanthoxylum, Sichuan pepper fruit
Chuan lian zi	*Meliae toosendan fructus*	Melia fruit
Chuan mu xiang	*Vladimiriae radix*	Vladimiria root
Chuan niu xi	*Cyathulae radix*	Sichuan ox knee root
Chuan xin lian	*Andrographitis paniculatae herba*	Kariyat; Green chiretta
Chuan xiong	*Ligustici chuanxiong radix*	Szechuan lovage root
Chuan xiong	*Ligustici chuanxiong radix*	Cnidium, Szechuan lovage root
Da huang	*Rhei radix et rhizoma*	Rhubarb root
Da huang	*Rhei rhizoma*	Rhubarb
Da huang	*Rhei radix et rhizoma*	Rhubarb root
Da qing ye	*Daqingye folium*	Isatis leaf, Woad leaf
Da suan	*Allii savtivi bulbus*	Garlic bulb
Da zao	*Ziziphi jujubae fructus*	Red date, Jujube fruit
Dai zhe shi	*Haematitum*	Hematite, Iron ore
Dan dou chi	*Sojae praeparatum semen*	Soybean prepared
Dan shen	*Salviae miltiorrhizae radix*	Salvia root
Dan zhu ye	*Lophatheri gracilis herba*	Bamboo leaf
Dang gui	*Angelicae sinensis radix*	Tang kuei root
Dang gui tou	*Angelicae sinensis caput radicis*	Tang kuei head
Dang gui wei	*Angelicae sinensis extremas radicis*	Tang kuei tail
Deng shen	*Codonopsis pilosulae radix*	Codonopsis root
Deng xin cao	*Junci effuse medulla*	Rush pith
Di gu pi	*Lycii chinensis radicis cortex*	Wolfberry root cortex

Pin Yin	Pharmaceutical	Common Name
Di long	*Lumbricus*	Earthworm
Di yu	*Sanguisorbae off icinalis radix*	Burnet-bloodwort root
Din jiao	*Gentianae macrophyllae radix*	Gentians root
Dong chong xia cao	*Cordyceps sinensis*	Cordyceps
Dong gua zi	*Benincasae semen*	Benincasa
Dong ling cao	*Rabdosia rucescens*	Rabdosia
Du huo	*Angelicae pubescentis radix*	Angelica root pubescent
Du huo	*Duhuo radix*	Angelica Duhuo root
Du zhong	*Eucommiae ulmoidis cortex*	Eucommia bark
Duan long gu	*Os draconis*	Dragon bone calcined, Fossilied bone calcined
Duan mu li	*Concha ostreae*	Oyster shell calcined
E jiao	*Asini cori gelatinum*	Donkey hide gelatin, Ass skin glue
E zhu	*Curcumae rhizoma*	Zedoary rhizome, Tumeric rhizome
Er cha	*Acacia seu uncaria pasta*	Black or white cutch paste
Fan xie ye	*Sennae folium*	Senna leaf
Fang feng	*Ledebouriellae divaricatae radix*	Siler root
Feng mi	*Mel*	Honey
Fo shou	*Citri sarcodactylis fructus*	Finger citron fruit
Fu hai shi	*Pumice*	Pumice
Fu ling	*Poriae cocos sclerotium*	Hoelen, Tuckahoe
Fu ling pi	*Poriae cocos cortex*	Tuckahoe skin
Fu pen zi	*Rubi fructus*	Chinese raspberry
Fu shen	*Poriae cocos sclerotium pararadicis*	Tuckahoe spirit
Fu zi (hei)	*Lateralis aconiti carmichaeli radix praeparata*	Prepared sichuan aconite root
Gan cao	*Glycyrrhizae uralensis radix*	Licorice root
Gan jiang	*Zingiberis officinalis rhizoma*	Dried ginger rhizome
Gan sui	*Euphorbiae kansui radix*	Kansui spurge root
Gao ben	*Ligustici rhizoma et radix*	Ligusticum root, Chinese lovage root
Gao liang jiang	*Alpiniae officinari rizoma*	Lesser galangal rhizome
Ge gen	*Puerariae radix*	Kudzu root
Ge hua	*Puerariae flos*	Pueraria flower

Pin Yin	**Pharmaceutical**	**Common Name**
Ge jie	*Gekko*	Gecko lizard
Gou qi zi	*Lycii chinensis fructus*	Lycium berry, Wolfberry fruit
Gou teng	*Uncariae cum uncis ramulus*	Gambir stem and hooks
Gu sui bu	*Drynariae fortunei rhizoma*	Drynaria rhizome
Gu ya	*Oryzae sativae germinantus fructus*	Rice sprout
Gua di	*Cucumeris pedicellus*	Melon pedicle
Gua lou	*Trichosanthis fructus*	Snakegourd fruit
Gua lou gen	*Trichosanthis radix*	Tricosanthes root
Gua lou pi	*Trichosanthis pericarpium*	Snakegourd peel
Gua lou ren	*Trichosanthis semen*	Snakegourd seed
Guan gui	*Cinnamomi cassiae cortex tubiformis*	Thin cinnamon bark form young trees
Guan ye liao	*Polygoni perfoliati herba*	Polygonum
Guang qin qian cao	*Desmodium styracifolium herba*	Desmodium herb
Gui zhi	*Cinnamomi cassiae ramulus*	Cinnamon twig
Hai dai	*Laminaria japonicae herba*	Algae
Hai feng teng	*Piperis futokadsurae calulis*	Kadsura stem
Hai jin sha	*Lygodii japonici herba*	Lygodium spores
Han fang ji	*Stephaniae tetrandrae radix*	Stephania root
Han lian cao	*Ecliptae prostratae herba*	Eclipta
Han sui shi	*Calcitum*	Calcite
He huan hua	*Albizziae julibrissin flos*	Mimosa tree flower, Silk tree flower
He shou wu	*Polygoni multiflori radix*	Fo ti root, Fleece flower root
He ye	*Nelumbinis nuciferae folium*	Lotus leaf
Hong hua	*Carthami tinctorii flos*	Safflower flower
Hong jing tian	*Rhodiola herba*	Rhodioia herb
Hong mao wu jia	*Acanthopanacis giraldii herba cortex*	Acanthopanacis stem bark
Hou po	*Magnoliae officinalis cortex*	Magnolia bark
Hou po hua	*Magnoliae flos*	Magnolia flower
Hu jiao	*Piperis nigris fructus*	Black pepper fruit
Hu ma ren	*Sesami radix*	Sesame
Hu po	*Succinum*	Amber
Hua shi	*Talcum*	Talc, Soapstone

Pin Yin	Pharmaceutical	Common Name
Hua shi cao	*Orthosiphon herba*	Orthosiphon herb
Huai hua mi	*Sophorae japonicae immaturus flos*	Pagoda tree flower bud
Huai jiao	*Sophorae japonicae fructus*	Pagoda tree fruit
Huai nui xi	*Achyranthis bidentatae radix*	Achyranthes root
Huang bai	*Phellodendri cortex*	Amur cork-tree bark
Huang jin	*Aurum*	Gold
Huang jing	*Polygonati rhizome*	Siberian Solomon seal rhizome
Huang lian	*Coptidis rhizoma*	Coptis rhizome
Huang qi	*Astragali membranaceus radix*	Astragalus Root, Yellow milk-vetch root
Huang qin	*Scutellariae baicalensis radix*	Skullcap root, Scute
Huang yao zi	*Dioscoreae bulbiferae tuber*	Dioscorea tuber
Huo xiang	*Agastaches seu pogostemi herba*	Patchouli, Agastache
Ji guan hua	*Celosiae cristatae flos*	Cockscomb flower
Ji lin shen	*Ginseng radix*	Panax ginseng, Jilin wild ginseng
Ji ning	*Salviae plebeya herba*	Salvia
Ji xue teng	*Jixueteng radix et caulis*	Millettia root and vine, Chicken blood vine
Jiang huang	*Curcumae rhizoma*	Turmeric rhizome
Jiao mu (chuan)	*Zanthoxyli bungeani semen*	Sichuan pepper seed
Jiao yi	*Saccharum granorum*	Maltose
Jie geng (ku)	*Platycodi grandiflori radix*	Balloon flower root, Platycodon
Jin yin hua	*Lonicerae japonicae flos*	Honeysuckle Flower
Jin yin teng	*Lonicerae japonicae ramus*	Honeysuckle stem
Jing jie	*Schizonepetae tenuifoliae herba seu flos*	Schizonepeta stem or bud
Jing mi	*Oryzae sativae semen*	Rice grain
Jiu jie chang pu	*Anemoni attaicae rhizomae*	Altaica rhizome, Anemone
Ju he	*Citri reticulatae semen*	Tangerine seed
Ju hong	*Citri erythrocarpae pericarpium*	Red tangerine peel
Ju hua	*Chrysanthemi morifolii flos*	Chrysanthemum fower
Jue ming zi	*Cassiae torae semen*	Cassia seeds

Pin Yin	Pharmaceutical	Common Name
Ku shen	Sophorae flavescentis radix	Sophora Root, Bitter ginseng root
Kuan dong hua	Tussilaginis farfarae flos	Coltsfoot flower
Kun bu	Algae thallus	Kelp thallus, Laminaria, Kombu thallus
Lai fu zi	Raphani sativi semen	Radish seed
Lian qiao	Forsythiae fructus	Forsythia fruit
Lian xu	Nelumbinis nuciferae stamen	Lotus stemen
Lian zi	Nelumbinis nuciferae semen	Lotus seed
Ling zhi	Ganoderma lucidum	Ganoderma
Liu huang	Sulphur	Sulphur
Long chi	Draconis dens	Dragons tooth, Fossilized tooth
Long dan cao	Gentianae longdancao radix	Gentian root
Long gu	Os draconis	Dragon bone
Long yan rou	Longanae arillus euphoriae	Longan fruit
Lu cha	Camella sinensis li	Green tea leaf
Lu dou	Phaseoli radiati semen	Mung bean
Lu gen	Phragmitis communis rhizoma	Reed rhizome
Lu jiao	Cornu cervi	Antler, Deerhorn
Luo Han Guo	Fructus Momordicae Grosvenori	Momordica Fruit
Luo shi teng	Tracachelospermi jasminoidis caulis	Star jasmine stem
Ma bian cao	Verbenae herba	Vervain leaf
Ma huang	Epherdrae herba	Ephedra
Mai men dong	Ophiopogonis japonici tuber	Ophiopogon tuber, Creeping lily-turf tuber
Mai ya	Hordei valgaria germinantus fructus	Barley sprout
Man jing zi	Viticis fructus	Vitex fruit
Man shan hong	Rhodod foliumendri	Rhododendron leaf
Mang xiao	Mirabilitum	Mirabilite, Glauber's salt
Mao dong qing	Ilicis pubescendis radix	Ilex root
Meng chong	Tabani Bivittati	Gadfly
Mo yao	Myrrha	Myrrh
Mu dan pi	Moutan radicis cortex	Tree peony root-bark
Mu jin hua	Hibisci Flos	Hibiscus flower
Mu li	Ostreae concha	Oyster shell

Pin Yin	Pharmaceutical	Common Name
Mu tong	Mutong caulis	Akebia stem
Mu xiang	Natrium sulphuricum	Saussurea
Niu bang zi	Arctii lappae fructus	Burdock fruit
Niu xi	Achyranthis bidentatae radix	Ox knee
Nu zhen zi	Ligustri lucidi fructus	Ligustrum fruit
Pi pa ye	Eriobotryae japonicae folium	Loquat leaf
Qian hu	Peucedani radix	Hogfennel root, Peucedanum
Qian niu zi	Pharbitidis semen	Cowherd seed
Qiang huo	Notopterygii rhizoma et radix	Notopterygium rhizome and root
Qin jiao	Gentianae qinjiao radix	Large-leaf gentian root
Qing hao	Artemisiae annuae herba	Artemesia, Sweet wormwood
Qing pi	Citri reticulatae viride pericarpium	Green (immature) tangerine peel
Qu mai	Dianthi herba	Dianthus, Pink flower herb
Ren gong niu huang	Calculus artificialis	Bos, cow gallstone
Ren shen	Ginseng radix	Ginseng root
Ren shen hong	Ginseng radix	Panax ginseng root (steamed until red)
Ren shen lu	Gensing cervix	Gensing root neck
Ren shen ye	Gensing folium	Gensing leaf
Rou cong rong	Cistanches deserticolae herba	Cistanche, Broomrape fleshy stem
Rou gui	Cinnamomi cassiae cortex	Cinnamon bark
Ru xiang	Olibanum gummi	Frankincense gum-resin
San leng	Sparganii rhizoma	Bur-reed rhizome
San qi, (Tian qi)	Pseudoginseng radix	Pseudoginseng root, notoginseng root
Sang bai pi	Mori albae radicis cortex	Morus bark, mulberry rootbark
Sang ji sheng	Loranthi ramulus	Loranthus stem
Sang ji sheng	Sangjisheng ramulus	Loranthus branches
Sang ji sheng	Sangjisheng ramulus	Mulberry mistletoe stems, loranthus
Sang piao xiao	Mantidis ootheca	Praying mantis egg case

Pin Yin	Pharmaceutical	Common Name
Sang shen	*Mori albae fructus*	Mulberry fruit bud
Sang ye	*Mori albae florium*	Mulberry leaf
Sang zhi	*Mori albae ramulus*	Mulberry twig
Sha ren	*Amomi fructus*	Cardamon fruit, Grains of paradise fruit or seeds
Sha yuan ji li	*Astragali complanati semen*	Astragalus, Flattened milk-vetch seed
Shan dou gen	*Sophorae tokinensis radix*	Sophora, Pigeon pea root
Shan yao	*Dioscoreae oppositae radix*	Wild yam
Shan zha	*Crataegi fructus*	Hawthorn unripe fruit
Shan zhu yu	*Corni officinalis fructus*	Dogwood fruit, Asiatic comelian cherry
Shao yao	*Paeoniae radix*	Peony
She chuang zi	*Cnidii monnieri fructus*	Cnidium seed
She shen	*Glehniae adenophorae seu radix*	Glehnia root
She xiang	*Moschus secretion*	Musk
Shen jin cao	*Lycopodii clavati herba*	Clubmoss
Shen qu	*Massa fermenta*	Medicated leaven
Sheng di huang	*Rehmanniae glutinosae radix*	Fresh rehmannia root, Chinese foxglove root
Sheng jiang	*Zingiberis officinalis recens rhizoma*	Fresh ginger root
Sheng ma	*Cimicifugae rhizoma*	Bugbane, Black Cohosh Rhizome, Cimicifuga
Shi chang pu	*Acori graminei rhizoma*	Acorus, Sweetflag rhizome
Shi gao	*Gypsum fibrosum*	Gypsum
Shi jue ming	*Concha haliotidis*	Abalone shell
Shi wei	*Pyrrosiae folium*	Pyrrosia leaf
Shu di huang	*Rehmanniae glutinosae conquitae radix*	Wine cooked rehmannia, Foxglove
Shu qi	*Dichroae Febrifugae Folium*	Dichroa leaf
Shui zhi	*Hirudo seu whitmania*	Leech
Su mu	*Sappan lignum*	Sappan heartwood
Su zi	*Perillae frutescentis fructus*	Perilla seed
Suan zao ren	*Zizyphi spinosae semen*	Zizyphus seed, Sour jujube
Suo sha	*Amoni semen*	Cardomon
Suo yang	*Cynomorii songaricii herba*	Cynomorium fleshy stem, Lock yang

Pin Yin	Pharmaceutical	Common Name
Tao ren	*Persicae semen*	Peach kernel
Tian hua fen	*Trichosanthis kirilowii radix*	Snakegourd root
Tian ji huang	*Hypericum perforatum*	St. john's wort
Tian ma	*Gastrodiae elatae rhizoma*	Gastrodia rhizome
Tian men dong	*Asparagi cochinchinensis tuber*	Chinese asparagus tuber
Tian zhu huang	*Bambusae textillis concretio silicea*	Siliceous secretions of bamboo
Tou gu cao	*Speranskia tuberculata*	Speranskia herb
Tu fu ling	*Smilacis glabrae rhizoma*	Smilax rhizome
Tu niu xi	*Achyranthis aspera radix*	Achyranthes root
Tu si zi	*Cuscutae chinensis semen*	Dodder seed
Wei ling xian	*Clematidis radix*	Clematis root
Wu jia shen	*Eleutherococci radix*	Eleuthero root
Wu mei	*Pruni mume*	Mume, Black plum fruit
Wu tou	*Aconiti radix*	Aconite root
Wu wei zi	*Schisandrae chinensis fructus*	Schisandra fruit
Wu yao	*Linderae strychnifoliae radix*	Lindera root
Wu zhu yu	*Evodiae rutaecarpae fructus*	Evodia fruit
Xi jiao	*Rhinoceri cornu*	Rhinoceros horn
Xi xin	*Asari herba radice*	Asarum, Chinese wild ginger
Xi yang shen	*Panacis quinquefolii radix*	American ginseng root
Xia ku cao	*Prunellae vulgaris spica*	Selfheal spike, Heal all spike
Xian he cao	*Agrimoniae pilosae herba*	Agrimony herb
Xian mao	*Curculiginis orchioidis rhizoma*	Curculigo rhizome, Golden eye-grass rhizome
Xiang fu	*Cyperi rotundi rhizoma*	Nut-grass rhizome, Cyperus
Xiang ru	*Elsholtziae seu moslae herba*	Aromatic madder
Xiao hui xiang	*Foeniculi vulgaris fructus*	Fennel fruit
Xie bai	*Allii bulbus macrostemi*	Bakeri, Chinese chive bulb
Xin yi hua	*Magnoliae liliflorae flos*	Magnolia flower
Xing ren	*Pruni armeniacae semen*	Apricot seed
Xiong dan	*Ursi vesica fellea*	Bear gallbladder

Pin Yin	**Pharmaceutical**	**Common Name**
Xiong huang	*Realgar*	Realgar, Arsenic disulfide
Xu duan	*Dipsaci radix*	Japanese teasel root
Xu sui zi	*Euphorbiae lathyridis semen*	Caper spurge seed, Moleplant seed
Xuan ming fen	*Mirabilitum purum*	Mirabilite, Sodium sulphate
Xuan shen	*Scrophulariae ningpoensis radix*	Scophularia root, Figwort root
Xue jie	*Draconis sanguis*	Dragon's blood resin
Yan hu suo	*Corydalis rhizome Yanhusuo*	Corydalis rhizome
Ye jiao teng	*Polygoni caulis multiflori*	Fleeceflower stem, Solomon's Seal Vine
Ye ju hua	*Chrysanthemi indici flos*	Wild Chrysanthemum flower
Ye shan shen	*Ginseng radix*	Wild ginseng
Yi mu cao	*Leonuri heterophylli herba*	Motherwort
Yi tang	*Saccharum granorrum*	Barley malt sugar
Yi yi ren	*Coicis lachryma-jobi*	Job's tears, Coxis
Yi zhi ren	*Alpiniae oxyphyllae fructus*	Alpinia fruit, Black cardamom
Yin chen hao	*Artemisiae yinchenhao herba*	Chinese wormwood
Yin guo ye	*Ginkgo bilobae folium*	Ginkgo leaf
Yin yang huo	*Epimedii herba*	Epimedium
You gua shi hu	*Ephemerantha fimbrata herba*	Ephemerantha herb
Yu jin	*Curcumae tuber*	Tumeric tuber
Yu xing cao	*Houttuyniae cordatae herba*	Houttuynia
Yu zhu	*Polygonati odorati rhizoma*	Solomon's Seal Rhizome, Polygonatum
Yuan Zhi	*Radix Polygalae Tenuifoliae*	Polygala Root
Zao jiao ci	*Gleditsiae chinensis spina*	Gleditsia thorn
Zao xiu	*Paridis rhizoma*	Paris rhizome
Ze xie	*Alismatis orientalis rhizoma*	Water plantain rhizome
Zhang nao	*Camphora*	Crystalized volatile oil of camphor
Zhe bei mu	*Fritillariae thunbergii bulbus*	Fritillaria bulb
Zhen zhu	*Margarita*	Pearl
Zhi can cao	*Glycyrrhizae Radix praeparata*	Honey-fried licorice root

Pin Yin	Pharmaceutical	Common Name
Zhi ke	*Citri aurantii fructus*	Bitter orange fruit
Zhi mu	*Anemarrhenae asphodeloidis radix*	Anemarrhena root
Zhi shi	*Citri seu ponciri immaturus fructus*	Immature bitter orange fruit
Zhi zi	*Gardenia jasminoidis fructus*	Gardenia fruit
Zhu li	*Bambusae succus*	Dried bamboo sap
Zhu ling	*Polypori umbellati sclerotium*	Polyporus
Zhu ru	*Bambusae in taenilis caulis*	Bamboo shavings
Zhu ye	*Bambusae folium*	Bamboo leaves
Zi cao	*Arnebiae seu lithospermi radix*	Lithospermum, Groomwell root
Zi hua di ding	*Violae cum radice herba*	Yedeon's Violet
Zi ran tong	*Pyritum*	Pyrite
Zi su ye	*Perillae frutescentis folium*	Perilla leaf
Zi su ye	*Perillae frutescentis folium*	Perilla leaf
Zi su zi	*Perillae frutescentis semen*	Perilla seed
Zi wan	*Asteris tatarici radix*	Purple aster root

Pharmaceutical (Herb List)

Pharmaceutical	Common Name	*Pin Yin*
Amomi cardamomi fructus	Cardamon fruit	*Bai dou kou*
Amomi kravanh fructus	Cardamon white	*Bai dou kou*
Angelicae dahurica radix	Angelica root	*Bai zhi*
Arecae catechu semen	Areca seed, Betel nut	*Bing lang*
Artemisiae argyi folium	Mugwort leaf	*Ai ye*
Atractylodis macrocephalae rhizoma	White Atractylodes root	*Bai zhu*
Atractylodis rizoma	Atractylodes rhizome	*Cang zhu*
Atractylodis rizoma	Atractylodes rhizome (red)	*Cang zhu*
Benzoinum	Styrax benzoin processed resin	*An xi xiang*
Biotae orientalis cacumen	Biota leaf	*Ce bai ye*
Biotae orientalis semen	Biota seed	*Bai zi ren*
Bombycis mori excrementum	Silkworm feces	*Can sha*
Broussonetie fructus	Broussonetia fruit	*Chu shi zi*
Bupleuri radix	Bupleurum root	*Chai hu*
Camelliae folium	Tea	*Cha ye*
Citri reticulatae pericarpium	Tangerine peel	*Chen pi*
Croton tiglii semen	Croton seed	*Ba dou*
Dictamni dasycarpi radicis cortex	Dittany root bark	*Bai xian pi*
Dioscorae hypoglaucae rhizome	Tokoro, Yam rhizome	*Bei xie*
Fritillariae bulbus	Fritillaria	*Bei mu*
Ginkgo bilobae semen	Ginkgo seed	*Bai guo*
Imperatae cylindricae rhizoma	Imperata rhizome	*Bai mao gen*
Isatidis seu baphicacanthi radix	Woad root	*Ban lan gen*
Lilii bulbus	Lily bulb	*Bai he*
Mentha herba	Mentha	*Bo he*
Menthae haplocalycis herba	Mint	*Bo he*
Menthae herba	Field Mint	*Bo he*
Morindae officinalis radix	Morinda root	*Ba ji tian*
Oldenlandiae diffusae herba	Oldenlandia	*Bai hua she she cao*
Paeoniae lactiflorae radix	White Peony root	*Bai shao*
Paeoniae rubra radix	Red peony root	*Chi shao*

Patriniae heterophyllae herba	Thiaspi, Patrinia	*Bai jiang cao*
Phaseoli calcarati semen	Aduki bean	*Chi xiao dou*
Pinellia tuber	Pinellia	*Ban xia*
Pinelliae tematae rhizome	Prepared Pinellia rhizome	*Ban xia (sheng)*
Pinelliae ternatae rhizoma	Pinellia rhizome	*Ban xia (fa)*
Plantaginis semen	Plantago seed	*Che qian zi*
Psoraleae corylifoliae fructus	Scuffy Pea	*Bu gu zhi*
Pulsatillae chinensis radix	Pulsatilla root	*Bai tou weng*
Smilacis china rizoma	Smilax rhizome	*Ba qia*
Tribuli terrestris fructus	Caltrop fruit	*Bai ji li*
Xanthii fructus	Xanthium, Cocklebur fruit	*Cang er zi*

Pharmaceutical	Common Name	Pin Yin
Fritillariae cirrhosae bulbus	Fritillaria bulb	*Chuan bei mu*
Zanthoxyli pericarpium bungeani	Zanthoxylum, Sichuan pepper fruit	*Chuan jiao*
Meliae toosendan fructus	Melia fruit	*Chuan lian zi*
Vladimiriae radix	Vladimiria root	*Chuan mu xiang*
Cyathulae radix	Sichuan ox knee root	*Chuan niu xi*
Andrographitis paniculatae herba	Kariyat; Green chiretta	*Chuan xin lian*
Ligustici chuanxiong radix	Szechuan lovage root	*Chuan xiong*
Ligustici chuanxiong radix	Cnidium, Szechuan lovage root	*Chuan xiong*
Rhei radix et rhizoma	Rhubarb root	*Da huang*
Rhei rhizoma	Rhubarb	*Da huang*
Rhei radix et rhizoma	Rhubarb root	*Da huang*
Daqingye folium	Isatis leaf, Woad leaf	*Da qing ye*
Allii savtivi bulbus	Garlic bulb	*Da suan*
Ziziphi jujubae fructus	Red date, Jujube fruit	*Da zao*
Haematitum	Hematite, Iron ore	*Dai zhe shi*
Sojae praeparatum semen	Soybean prepared	*Dan dou chi*
Salviae miltiorrhizae radix	Salvia root	*Dan shen*
Lophatheri gracilis herba	Bamboo leaf	*Dan zhu ye*
Angelicae sinensis radix	Tang kuei root	*Dang gui*
Angelicae sinensis caput radicis	Tang kuei head	*Dang gui tou*
Angelicae sinensis extremas radicis	Tang kuei tail	*Dang gui wei*
Codonopsis pilosulae radix	Codonopsis root	*Deng shen*
Junci effuse medulla	Rush pith	*Deng xin cao*
Lycii chinensis radicis cortex	Wolfberry root cortex	*Di gu pi*
Lumbricus	Earthworm	*Di long*
Sanguisorbae off icinalis radix	Burnet-bloodwort root	*Di yu*
Gentianae macrophyllae radix	Gentians root	*Din jiao*
Cordyceps sinensis	Cordyceps	*Dong chong xia cao*
Benincasae semen	Benincasa	*Dong gua zi*
Rabdosia rucescens	Rabdosia	*Dong ling cao*
Angelicae pubescentis radix	Angelica root pubescent	*Du huo*
Duhuo radix	Angelica Duhuo root	*Du huo*

Eucommiae ulmoidis cortex	Eucommia bark	*Du zhong*
Os draconis	Dragon bone calcined, Fossilied bone calcined	*Duan long gu*
Concha ostreae	Oyster shell calcined	*Duan mu li*
Asini cori gelatinum	Donkey hide gelatin, Ass skin glue	*E jiao*
Curcumae rhizoma	Zedoary rhizome, Tumeric rhizome	*E zhu*
Acacia seu uncaria pasta	Black or white cutch paste	*Er cha*
Sennae folium	Senna leaf	*Fan xie ye*
Ledebouriellae divaricatae radix	Siler root	*Fang feng*

Pharmaceutical	Common Name	*Pin Yin*
Mel	Honey	*Feng mi*
Citri sarcodactylis fructus	Finger citron fruit	*Fo shou*
Pumice	Pumice	*Fu hai shi*
Poriae cocos sclerotium	Hoelen, Tuckahoe	*Fu ling*
Poriae cocos cortex	Tuckahoe skin	*Fu ling pi*
Rubi fructus	Chinese raspberry	*Fu pen zi*
Poriae cocos sclerotium pararadicis	Tuckahoe spirit	*Fu shen*
Lateralis aconiti carmichaeli radix praeparata	Prepared sichuan aconite root	*Fu zi (hei)*
Glycyrrhizae uralensis radix	Licorice root	*Gan cao*
Zingiberis officinalis rhizoma	Dried ginger rhizome	*Gan jiang*
Euphorbiae kansui radix	Kansui spurge root	*Gan sui*
Ligustici rhizoma et radix	Ligusticum root, Chinese lovage root	*Gao ben*
Alpiniae officinari rizoma	Lesser galangal rhizome	*Gao liang jiang*
Puerariae radix	Kudzu root	*Ge gen*
Puerariae flos	Pueraria flower	*Ge hua*
Gekko	Gecko lizard	*Ge jie*
Lycii chinensis fructus	Lycium berry, Wolfberry fruit	*Gou qi zi*
Uncariae cum uncis ramulus	Gambir stem and hooks	*Gou teng*
Drynariae fortunei rhizoma	Drynaria rhizome	*Gu sui bu*
Oryzae sativae germinantus fructus	Rice sprout	*Gu ya*
Cucumeris pedicellus	Melon pedicle	*Gua di*
Trichosanthis fructus	Snakegourd fruit	*Gua lou*
Trichosanthis radix	Tricosanthes root	*Gua lou gen*
Trichosanthis pericarpium	Snakegourd peel	*Gua lou pi*
Trichosanthis semen	Snakegourd seed	*Gua lou ren*
Cinnamomi cassiae cortex tubiformis	Thin cinnamon bark form young trees	*Guan gui*
Polygoni perfoliati herba	Polygonum	*Guan ye liao*
Desmodium styracifolium herba	Desmodium herb	*Guang qin qian cao*
Cinnamomi cassiae ramulus	Cinnamon twig	*Gui zhi*
Laminaria japonicae herba	Algae	*Hai dai*

Piperis futokadsurae calulis	Kadsura stem	*Hai feng teng*
Lygodii japonici herba	Lygodium spores	*Hai jin sha*
Stephaniae tetrandrae radix	Stephania root	*Han fang ji*
Ecliptae prostratae herba	Eclipta	*Han lian cao*
Calcitum	Calcite	*Han sui shi*
Albizziae julibrissin flos	Mimosa tree flower, Silk tree flower	*He huan hua*
Polygoni multiflori radix	Fo ti root, Fleece flower root	*He shou wu*
Nelumbinis nuciferae folium	Lotus leaf	*He ye*
Carthami tinctorii flos	Safflower flower	*Hong hua*
Rhodiola herba	Rhodioia herb	*Hong jing tian*

Pharmaceutical	Common Name	Pin Yin
Acanthopanacis giraldii herba cortex	Acanthopanacis stem bark	*Hong mao wu jia*
Magnoliae officinalis cortex	Magnolia bark	*Hou po*
Magnoliae flos	Magnolia flower	*Hou po hua*
Piperis nigris fructus	Black pepper fruit	*Hu jiao*
Sesami radix	Sesame	*Hu ma ren*
Succinum	Amber	*Hu po*
Talcum	Talc, Soapstone	*Hua shi*
Orthosiphon herba	Orthosiphon herb	*Hua shi cao*
Sophorae japonicae immaturus flos	Pagoda tree flower bud	*Huai hua mi*
Sophorae japonicae fructus	Pagoda tree fruit	*Huai jiao*
Achyranthis bidentatae radix	Achyranthes root	*Huai nui xi*
Phellodendri cortex	Amur cork-tree bark	*Huang bai*
Aurum	Gold	*Huang jin*
Polygonati rhizome	Siberian Solomon seal rhizome	*Huang jing*
Coptidis rhizoma	Coptis rhizome	*Huang lian*
Astragali membranaceus radix	Astragalus Root, Yellow milk-vetch root	*Huang qi*
Scutellariae baicalensis radix	Skullcap root, Scute	*Huang qin*
Dioscoreae bulbiferae tuber	Dioscorea tuber	*Huang yao zi*
Agastaches seu pogostemi herba	Patchouli, Agastache	*Huo xiang*
Celosiae cristatae flos	Cockscomb flower	*Ji guan hua*
Ginseng radix	Panax ginseng, Jilin wild ginseng	*Ji lin shen*
Salviae plebeya herba	Salvia	*Ji ning*
Jixueteng radix et caulis	Millettia root and vine, Chicken blood vine	*Ji xue teng*
Curcumae rhizoma	Turmeric rhizome	*Jiang huang*
Zanthoxyli bungeani semen	Sichuan pepper seed	*Jiao mu (chuan)*
Saccharum granorum	Maltose	*Jiao yi*
Platycodi grandiflori radix	Balloon flower root, Platycodon	*Jie geng (ku)*
Lonicerae japonicae flos	Honeysuckle Flower	*Jin yin hua*
Lonicerae japonicae ramus	Honeysuckle stem	*Jin yin teng*

Schizonepetae tenuifoliae herba seu flos	Schizonepeta stem or bud	*Jing jie*
Oryzae sativae semen	Rice grain	*Jing mi*
Anemoni attaicae rhizomae	Altaica rhizome, Anemone	*Jiu jie chang pu*
Citri reticulatae semen	Tangerine seed	*Ju he*
Citri erythrocarpae pericarpium	Red tangerine peel	*Ju hong*
Chrysanthemi morifolii flos	Chrysanthemum fower	*Ju hua*
Cassiae torae semen	Cassia seeds	*Jue ming zi*
Sophorae flavescentis radix	Sophora Root, Bitter ginseng root	*Ku shen*
Tussilaginis farfarae flos	Coltsfoot flower	*Kuan dong hua*

Pharmaceutical	Common Name	Pin Yin
Algae thallus	Kelp thallus, Laminaria, Kombu thallus	*Kun bu*
Raphani sativi semen	Radish seed	*Lai fu zi*
Forsythiae fructus	Forsythia fruit	*Lian qiao*
Nelumbinis nuciferae stamen	Lotus stemen	*Lian xu*
Nelumbinis nuciferae semen	Lotus seed	*Lian zi*
Ganoderma lucidum	Ganoderma	*Ling zhi*
Sulphur	Sulphur	*Liu huang*
Draconis dens	Dragons tooth, Fossilized tooth	*Long chi*
Gentianae longdancao radix	Gentian root	*Long dan cao*
Os draconis	Dragon bone	*Long gu*
Longanae arillus euphoriae	Longan fruit	*Long yan rou*
Camella sinensis li	Green tea leaf	*Lu cha*
Phaseoli radiati semen	Mung bean	*Lu dou*
Phragmitis communis rhizoma	Reed rhizome	*Lu gen*
Comu cervi	Antler, Deerhorn	*Lu jiao*
Fructus Momordicae Grosvenori	Momordica Fruit	*Luo Han Guo*
Tracachelospermi jasminoidis caulis	Star jasmine stem	*Luo shi teng*
Verbenae herba	Vervain leaf	*Ma bian cao*
Epherdrae herba	Ephedra	*Ma huang*
Ophiopogonis japonici tuber	Ophiopogon tuber, Creeping lily-turf tuber	*Mai men dong*
Hordei valgaria germinantus fructus	Barley sprout	*Mai ya*
Viticis fructus	Vitex fruit	*Man jing zi*
Rhodod foliumendri	Rhododendron leaf	*Man shan hong*
Mirabilitum	Mirabilite, Glauber's salt	*Mang xiao*
Ilicis pubescendis radix	Ilex root	*Mao dong qing*
Tabani Bivittati	Gadfly	*Meng chong*
Myrrha	Myrrh	*Mo yao*
Moutan radicis cortex	Tree peony root-bark	*Mu dan pi*
Hibisci Flos	Hibiscus flower	*Mu jin hua*
Ostreae concha	Oyster shell	*Mu li*
Mutong caulis	Akebia stem	*Mu tong*

Natrium sulphuricum	Saussurea	*Mu xiang*
Arctii lappae fructus	Burdock fruit	*Niu bang zi*
Achyranthis bidentatae radix	Ox knee	*Niu xi*
Ligustri lucidi fructus	Ligustrum fruit	*Nu zhen zi*
Eriobotryae japonicae folium	Loquat leaf	*Pi pa ye*
Peucedani radix	Hogfennel root, Peucedanum	*Qian hu*
Pharbitidis semen	Cowherd seed	*Qian niu zi*
Notopterygii rhizoma et radix	Notopterygium rhizome and root	*Qiang huo*
Gentianae qinjiao radix	Large-leaf gentian root	*Qin jiao*

Pharmaceutical	Common Name	*Pin Yin*
Artemisiae annuae herba	Artemesia, Sweet wormwood	*Qing hao*
Citri reticulatae viride pericarpium	Green (immature) tangerine peel	*Qing pi*
Dianthi herba	Dianthus, Pink flower herb	*Qu mai*
Calculus artificialis	Bos, cow gallstone	*Ren gong niu huang*
Ginseng radix	Ginseng root	*Ren shen*
Ginseng radix	Panax ginseng root (steamed until red)	*Ren shen hong*
Gensing cervix	Gensing root neck	*Ren shen lu*
Gensing folium	Gensing leaf	*Ren shen ye*
Cistanches deserticolae herba	Cistanche, Broomrape fleshy stem	*Rou cong rong*
Cinnamomi cassiae cortex	Cinnamon bark	*Rou gui*
Olibanum gummi	Frankincense gum-resin	*Ru xiang*
Sparganii rhizoma	Bur-reed rhizome	*San leng*
Pseudoginseng radix	Pseudoginseng root, notoginseng root	*San qi, (Tian qi)*
Mori albae radicis cortex	Morus bark, mulberry rootbark	*Sang bai pi*
Loranthi ramulus	Loranthus stem	*Sang ji sheng*
Sangjisheng ramulus	Loranthus branches	*Sang ji sheng*
Sangjisheng ramulus	Mulberry mistletoe stems, loranthus	*Sang ji sheng*
Mantidis ootheca	Praying mantis egg case	*Sang piao xiao*
Mori albae fructus	Mulberry fruit bud	*Sang shen*
Mori albae florium	Mulberry leaf	*Sang ye*
Mori albae ramulus	Mulberry twig	*Sang zhi*
Amomi fructus	Cardamon fruit, Grains of paradise fruit or seeds	*Sha ren*
Astragali complanati semen	Astragalus, Flattened milk-vetch seed	*Sha yuan ji li*
Sophorae tokinensis radix	Sophora, Pigeon pea root	*Shan dou gen*
Dioscoreae oppositae radix	Wild yam	*Shan yao*
Crataegi fructus	Hawthorn unripe fruit	*Shan zha*
Comi officinalis fructus	Dogwood fruit, Asiatic comelian cherry	*Shan zhu yu*

Paeoniae radix	Peony	Shao yao
Cnidii monnieri fructus	Cnidium seed	She chuang zi
Glehniae adenophorae seu radix	Glehnia root	She shen
Moschus secretion	Musk	She xiang
Lycopodii clavati herba	Clubmoss	Shen jin cao
Massa fermenta	Medicated leaven	Shen qu
Rehmanniae glutinosae radix	Fresh rehmannia root, Chinese foxglove root	Sheng di huang

Pharmaceutical	Common Name	*Pin Yin*
Zingiberis officinalis recens rhizoma	Fresh ginger root	*Sheng jiang*
Cimicifugae rhizoma	Bugbane, Black Cohosh Rhizome, Cimicifuga	*Sheng ma*
Acori graminei rhizoma	Acorus, Sweetflag rhizome	*Shi chang pu*
Gypsum fibrosum	Gypsum	*Shi gao*
Concha haliotidis	Abalone shell	*Shi jue ming*
Pyrrosiae folium	Pyrrosia leaf	*Shi wei*
Rehmanniae glutinosae conquitae radix	Wine cooked rehmannia, Foxglove	*Shu di huang*
Dichroae Febrifugae Folium	Dichroa leaf	*Shu qi*
Hirudo seu whitmania	Leech	*Shui zhi*
Sappan lignum	Sappan heartwood	*Su mu*
Perillae frutescentis fructus	Perilla seed	*Su zi*
Zizyphi spinosae semen	Zizyphus seed, Sour jujube	*Suan zao ren*
Amoni semen	Cardomon	*Suo sha*
Cynomorii songaricii herba	Cynomorium fleshy stem, Lock yang	*Suo yang*
Persicae semen	Peach kernel	*Tao ren*
Trichosanthis kirilowii radix	Snakegourd root	*Tian hua fen*
Hypericum perforatum	St. john's wort	*Tian ji huang*
Gastrodiae elatae rhizoma	Gastrodia rhizome	*Tian ma*
Asparagi cochinchinensis tuber	Chinese asparagus tuber	*Tian men dong*
Bambusae textillis concretio silicea	Siliceous secretions of bamboo	*Tian zhu huang*
Speranskia tuberculata	Speranskia herb	*Tou gu cao*
Smilacis glabrae rhizoma	Smilax rhizome	*Tu fu ling*
Achyranthis aspera radix	Achyranthes root	*Tu niu xi*
Cuscutae chinensis semen	Dodder seed	*Tu si zi*
Clematidis radix	Clematis root	*Wei ling xian*
Eleutherococci radix	Eleuthero root	*Wu jia shen*
Pruni mume	Mume, Black plum fruit	*Wu mei*
Aconiti radix	Aconite root	*Wu tou*
Schisandrae chinensis fructus	Schisandra fruit	*Wu wei zi*
Linderae strychnifoliae radix	Lindera root	*Wu yao*
Evodiae rutaecarpae fructus	Evodia fruit	*Wu zhu yu*

Rhinoceri cornu	Rhinoceros horn	*Xi jiao*
Asari herba radice	Asarum, Chinese wild ginger	*Xi xin*
Panacis quinquefolii radix	American ginseng root	*Xi yang shen*
Prunellae vulgaris spica	Selfheal spike, Heal all spike	*Xia ku cao*
Agrimoniae pilosae herba	Agrimony herb	*Xian he cao*
Curculiginis orchioidis rhizoma	Curculigo rhizome, Golden eye-grass rhizome	*Xian mao*
Cyperi rotundi rhizoma	Nut-grass rhizome, Cyperus	*Xiang fu*

Pharmaceutical	Common Name	Pin Yin
Elsholtziae seu moslae herba	Aromatic madder	*Xiang ru*
Foeniculi vulgaris fructus	Fennel fruit	*Xiao hui xiang*
Allii bulbus macrostemi	Bakeri, Chinese chive bulb	*Xie bai*
Magnoliae liliflorae flos	Magnolia flower	*Xin yi hua*
Pruni armeniacae semen	Apricot seed	*Xing ren*
Ursi vesica fellea	Bear gallbladder	*Xiong dan*
Realgar	Realgar, Arsenic disulfide	*Xiong huang*
Dipsaci radix	Japanese teasel root	*Xu duan*
Euphorbiae lathyridis semen	Caper spurge seed, Moleplant seed	*Xu sui zi*
Mirabilitum purum	Mirabilite, Sodium sulphate	*Xuan ming fen*
Scrophulariae ningpoensis radix	Scophularia root, Figwort root	*Xuan shen*
Draconis sanguis	Dragon's blood resin	*Xue jie*
Corydalis rhizome Yanhusuo	Corydalis rhizome	*Yan hu suo*
Polygoni caulis multiflori	Fleeceflower stem, Solomon's Seal Vine	*Ye jiao teng*
Chrysanthemi indici flos	Wild Chrysanthemum flower	*Ye ju hua*
Ginseng radix	Wild ginseng	*Ye shan shen*
Leonuri heterophylli herba	Motherwort	*Yi mu cao*
Saccharum granorrum	Barley malt sugar	*Yi tang*
Coicis lachryma-jobi	Job's tears, Coxis	*Yi yi ren*
Alpiniae oxyphyllae fructus	Alpinia fruit, Black cardamom	*Yi zhi ren*
Artemisiae yinchenhao herba	Chinese wormwood	*Yin chen hao*
Ginkgo bilobae folium	Ginkgo leaf	*Yin guo ye*
Epimedii herba	Epimedium	*Yin yang huo*
Ephemerantha fimbrata herba	Ephemerantha herb	*You gua shi hu*
Curcumae tuber	Tumeric tuber	*Yu jin*
Houttuyniae cordatae herba	Houttuynia	*Yu xing cao*
Polygonati odorati rhizoma	Solomon's Seal Rhizome, Polygonatum	*Yu zhu*
Radix Polygalae Tenuifoliae	Polygala Root	*Yuan Zhi*
Gleditsiae chinensis spina	Gleditsia thorn	*Zao jiao ci*

Paridis rhizoma	Paris rhizome	*Zao xiu*
Alismatis orientalis rhizoma	Water plantain rhizome	*Ze xie*
Camphora	Crystalized volatile oil of camphor	*Zhang nao*
Fritillariae thunbergii bulbus	Fritillaria bulb	*Zhe bei mu*
Margarita	Pearl	*Zhen zhu*
Glycyrrhizae Radix praeparata	Honey-fried licorice root	*Zhi can cao*
Citri aurantii fructus	Bitter orange fruit	*Zhi ke*
Anemarrhenae asphodeloidis radix	Anemarrhena root	*Zhi mu*
Citri seu ponciri immaturus fructus	Immature bitter orange fruit	*Zhi shi*
Gardenia jasminoidis fructus	Gardenia fruit	*Zhi zi*

Pharmaceutical	Common Name	*Pin Yin*
Bambusae succus	Dried bamboo sap	*Zhu li*
Polypori umbellati sclerotium	Polyporus	*Zhu ling*
Bambusae in taenilis caulis	Bamboo shavings	*Zhu ru*
Bambusae folium	Bamboo leaves	*Zhu ye*
Arnebiae seu lithospermi radix	Lithospermum, Groomwell root	*Zi cao*
Violae cum radice herba	Yedeon's Violet	*Zi hua di ding*
Pyritum	Pyrite	*Zi ran tong*
Perillae frutescentis folium	Perilla leaf	*Zi su ye*
Perillae frutescentis folium	Perilla leaf	*Zi su ye*
Perillae frutescentis semen	Perilla seed	*Zi su zi*
Asteris tatarici radix	Purple aster root	*Zi wan*

Common Name (Herb List)

Common Name	Pharmaceutical	*Pin Yin*
Abalone shell	*Concha haliotidis*	*Shi jue ming*
Acanthopanacis stem bark	*Acanthopanacis giraldii herba cortex*	*Hong mao wu jia*
Achyranthes root	*Achyranthis bidentatae radix*	*Huai nui xi*
Achyranthes root	*Achyranthis aspera radix*	*Tu niu xi*
Aconite root	*Aconiti radix*	*Wu tou*
Acorus, Sweetflag rhizome	*Acori graminei rhizoma*	*Shi chang pu*
Aduki bean	*Phaseoli calcarati semen*	*Chi xiao dou*
Agrimony herb	*Agrimoniae pilosae herba*	*Xian he cao*
Akebia stem	*Mutong caulis*	*Mu tong*
Algae	*Laminaria japonicae herba*	*Hai dai*
Alpinia fruit, Black cardamom	*Alpiniae oxyphyllae fructus*	*Yi zhi ren*
Altaica rhizome, Anemone	*Anemoni attaicae rhizomae*	*Jiu jie chang pu*
Amber	*Succinum*	*Hu po*
American ginseng root	*Panacis quinquefolii radix*	*Xi yang shen*
Amur cork-tree bark	*Phellodendri cortex*	*Huang bai*
Anemarrhena root	*Anemarrhenae asphodeloidis radix*	*Zhi mu*
Angelica Duhuo root	*Duhuo radix*	*Du huo*
Angelica root	*Angelicae dahurica radix*	*Bai zhi*
Angelica root pubescent	*Angelicae pubescentis radix*	*Du huo*
Antler, Deerhorn	*Cornu cervi*	*Lu jiao*
Apricot seed	*Pruni armeniacae semen*	*Xing ren*
Areca seed, Betel nut	*Arecae catechu semen*	*Bing lang*
Aromatic madder	*Elsholtziae seu moslae herba*	*Xiang ru*
Asarum, Chinese wild ginger	*Asari herba radice*	*Xi xin*
Artemesia, Sweet wormwood	*Artemisiae annuae herba*	*Qing hao*
Astragalus Root, Yellow milk-vetch root	*Astragali membranaceus radix*	*Huang qi*
Astragalus, Flattened milk-vetch seed	*Astragali complanati semen*	*Sha yuan ji li*
Atractylodes rhizome	*Atractylodis rizoma*	*Cang zhu*
Atractylodes rhizome (red)	*Atractylodis rizoma*	*Cang zhu*
Bakeri, Chinese chive bulb	*Allii bulbus macrostemi*	*Xie bai*

Common Name	Pharmaceutical	Pin Yin
Balloon flower root, Platycodon	*Platycodi grandiflori radix*	*Jie geng (ku)*
Bamboo leaf	*Lophatheri gracilis herba*	*Dan zhu ye*
Bamboo leaves	*Bambusae folium*	*Zhu ye*
Bamboo shavings	*Bambusae in taenilis caulis*	*Zhu ru*
Barley malt sugar	*Saccharum granorrum*	*Yi tang*
Barley sprout	*Hordei valgaria germinantus fructus*	*Mai ya*
Bear gallbladder	*Ursi vesica fellea*	*Xiong dan*
Benincasa	*Benincasae semen*	*Dong gua zi*
Biota leaf	*Biotae orientalis cacumen*	*Ce bai ye*
Biota seed	*Biotae orientalis semen*	*Bai zi ren*
Bitter orange fruit	*Citri aurantii fructus*	*Zhi ke*
Black or white cutch paste	*Acacia seu uncaria pasta*	*Er cha*
Black pepper fruit	*Piperis nigris fructus*	*Hu jiao*
Bos, cow gallstone	*Calculus artificialis*	*Ren gong niu huang*
Broussonetia fruit	*Broussonetie fructus*	*Chu shi zi*
Bugbane, Black Cohosh Rhizome, Cimicifuga	*Cimicifugae rhizoma*	*Sheng ma*
Bupleurum root	*Bupleuri radix*	*Chai hu*
Burdock fruit	*Arctii lappae fructus*	*Niu bang zi*
Burnet-bloodwort root	*Sanguisorbae off icinalis radix*	*Di yu*
Bur-reed rhizome	*Sparganii rhizoma*	*San leng*
Calcite	*Calcitum*	*Han sui shi*
Caltrop fruit	*Tribuli terrestris fructus*	*Bai ji li*
Caper spurge seed, Moleplant seed	*Euphorbiae lathyridis semen*	*Xu sui zi*
Cardamon fruit	*Amomi cardamomi fructus*	*Bai dou kou*
Cardamon fruit, Grains of paradise fruit or seeds	*Amomi fructus*	*Sha ren*
Cardamon white	*Amomi kravanh fructus*	*Bai dou kou*
Cardomon	*Amoni semen*	*Suo sha*
Cassia seeds	*Cassiae torae semen*	*Jue ming zi*
Chinese asparagus tuber	*Asparagi cochinchinensis tuber*	*Tian men dong*
Chinese raspberry	*Rubi fructus*	*Fu pen zi*

Common Name	Pharmaceutical	*Pin Yin*
Chinese wormwood	*Artemisiae yinchenhao herba*	*Yin chen hao*
Chrysanthemum fower	*Chrysanthemi morifolii flos*	*Ju hua*
Cinnamon bark	*Cinnamomi cassiae cortex*	*Rou gui*
Cinnamon twig	*Cinnamomi cassiae ramulus*	*Gui zhi*
Cistanche, Broomrape fleshy stem	*Cistanches deserticolae herba*	*Rou cong rong*
Clematis root	*Clematidis radix*	*Wei ling xian*
Clubmoss	*Lycopodii clavati herba*	*Shen jin cao*
Cnidium seed	*Cnidii monnieri fructus*	*She chuang zi*
Cnidium, Szechuan lovage root	*Ligustici chuanxiong radix*	*Chuan xiong*
Cockscomb flower	*Celosiae cristatae flos*	*Ji guan hua*
Codonopsis root	*Codonopsis pilosulae radix*	*Deng shen*
Coltsfoot flower	*Tussilaginis farfarae flos*	*Kuan dong hua*
Coptis rhizome	*Coptidis rhizoma*	*Huang lian*
Cordyceps	*Cordyceps sinensis*	*Dong chong xia cao*
Corydalis rhizome	*Corydalis rhizome Yanhusuo*	*Yan hu suo*
Cowherd seed	*Pharbitidis semen*	*Qian niu zi*
Croton seed	*Croton tiglii semen*	*Ba dou*
Crystalized volatile oil of camphor	*Camphora*	*Zhang nao*
Curculigo rhizome, Golden eye-grass rhizome	*Curculiginis orchioidis rhizoma*	*Xian mao*
Cynomorium fleshy stem, Lock yang	*Cynomorii songaricii herba*	*Suo yang*
Desmodium herb	*Desmodium styracifolium herba*	*Guang qin qian cao*
Dianthus, Pink flower herb	*Dianthi herba*	*Qu mai*
Dichroa leaf	*Dichroae Febrifugae Folium*	*Shu qi*
Dioscorea tuber	*Dioscoreae bulbiferae tuber*	*Huang yao zi*
Dittany root bark	*Dictamni dasycarpi radicis cortex*	*Bai xian pi*
Dodder seed	*Cuscutae chinensis semen*	*Tu si zi*
Dogwood fruit, Asiatic comelian cherry	*Comi officinalis fructus*	*Shan zhu yu*
Donkey hide gelatin, Ass skin glue	*Asini cori gelatinum*	*E jiao*

Common Name	Pharmaceutical	Pin Yin
Dragon bone	*Os draconis*	*Long gu*
Dragon bone calcined, Fossilied bone calcined	*Os draconis*	*Duan long gu*
Dragon's blood resin	*Draconis sanguis*	*Xue jie*
Dragons tooth, Fossilized tooth	*Draconis dens*	*Long chi*
Dried bamboo sap	*Bambusae succus*	*Zhu li*
Dried ginger rhizome	*Zingiberis officinalis rhizoma*	*Gan jiang*
Drynaria rhizome	*Drynariae fortunei rhizoma*	*Gu sui bu*
Earthworm	*Lumbricus*	*Di long*
Eclipta	*Ecliptae prostratae herba*	*Han lian cao*
Eleuthero root	*Eleutherococci radix*	*Wu jia shen*
Ephedra	*Epherdrae herba*	*Ma huang*
Ephemerantha herb	*Ephemerantha fimbrata herba*	*You gua shi hu*
Epimedium	*Epimedii herba*	*Yin yang huo*
Eucommia bark	*Eucommiae ulmoidis cortex*	*Du zhong*
Evodia fruit	*Evodiae rutaecarpae fructus*	*Wu zhu yu*
Fennel fruit	*Foeniculi vulgaris fructus*	*Xiao hui xiang*
Field Mint	*Menthae herba*	*Bo he*
Finger citron fruit	*Citri sarcodactylis fructus*	*Fo shou*
Fleeceflower stem, Solomon's Seal Vine	*Polygoni caulis multiflori*	*Ye jiao teng*
Fo ti root, Fleece flower root	*Polygoni multiflori radix*	*He shou wu*
Forsythia fruit	*Forsythiae fructus*	*Lian qiao*
Frankincense gum-resin	*Olibanum gummi*	*Ru xiang*
Fresh ginger root	*Zingiberis officinalis recens rhizoma*	*Sheng jiang*
Fresh rehmannia root, Chinese foxglove root	*Rehmanniae glutinosae radix*	*Sheng di huang*
Fritillaria	*Fritillariae bulbus*	*Bei mu*
Fritillaria bulb	*Fritillariae thunbergii bulbus*	*Zhe bei mu*
Fritillaria bulb	*Fritillariae cirrhosae bulbus*	*Chuan bei mu*
Gadfly	*Tabani Bivittati*	*Meng chong*
Gambir stem and hooks	*Uncariae cum uncis ramulus*	*Gou teng*
Ganoderma	*Ganoderma lucidum*	*Ling zhi*
Gardenia fruit	*Gardenia jasminoidis fructus*	*Zhi zi*

Common Name	Pharmaceutical	Pin Yin
Garlic bulb	*Allii sativi bulbus*	*Da suan*
Gastrodia rhizome	*Gastrodiae elatae rhizoma*	*Tian ma*
Gecko lizard	*Gekko*	*Ge jie*
Gensing leaf	*Gensing folium*	*Ren shen ye*
Gensing root neck	*Gensing cervix*	*Ren shen lu*
Gentian root	*Gentianae longdancao radix*	*Long dan cao*
Gentians root	*Gentianae macrophyllae radix*	*Din jiao*
Ginkgo leaf	*Ginkgo bilobae folium*	*Yin guo ye*
Ginkgo seed	*Ginkgo bilobae semen*	*Bai guo*
Ginseng root	*Ginseng radix*	*Ren shen*
Gleditsia thorn	*Gleditsiae chinensis spina*	*Zao jiao ci*
Glehnia root	*Glehniae adenophorae seu radix*	*She shen*
Gold	*Aurum*	*Huang jin*
Green (immature) tangerine peel	*Citri reticulatae viride pericarpium*	*Qing pi*
Green tea leaf	*Camella sinensis li*	*Lu cha*
Gypsum	*Gypsum fibrosum*	*Shi gao*
Hawthorn unripe fruit	*Crataegi fructus*	*Shan zha*
Hematite, Iron ore	*Haematitum*	*Dai zhe shi*
Hibiscus flower	*Hibisci Flos*	*Mu jin hua*
Hoelen, Tuckahoe	*Poriae cocos sclerotium*	*Fu ling*
Hogfennel root, Peucedanum	*Peucedani radix*	*Qian hu*
Honey	*Mel*	*Feng mi*
Honey-fried licorice root	*Glycyrrhizae Radix praeparata*	*Zhi can cao*
Honeysuckle Flower	*Lonicerae japonicae flos*	*Jin yin hua*
Honeysuckle stem	*Lonicerae japonicae ramus*	*Jin yin teng*
Houttuynia	*Houttuyniae cordatae herba*	*Yu xing cao*
Ilex root	*Ilicis pubescendis radix*	*Mao dong qing*
Immature bitter orange fruit	*Citri seu ponciri immaturus fructus*	*Zhi shi*
Imperata rhizome	*Imperatae cylindricae rhizoma*	*Bai mao gen*
Isatis leaf, Woad leaf	*Daqingye folium*	*Da qing ye*
Japanese teasel root	*Dipsaci radix*	*Xu duan*
Job's tears, Coxis	*Coicis lachryma-jobi*	*Yi yi ren*
Kadsura stem	*Piperis futokadsurae calulis*	*Hai feng teng*
Kansui spurge root	*Euphorbiae kansui radix*	*Gan sui*

Common Name	Pharmaceutical	*Pin Yin*
Kariyat; Green chiretta	*Andrographitis paniculatae herba*	*Chuan xin lian*
Kelp thallus, Laminaria, Kombu thallus	*Algae thallus*	*Kun bu*
Kudzu root	*Puerariae radix*	*Ge gen*
Large-leaf gentian root	*Gentianae qinjiao radix*	*Qin jiao*
Leech	*Hirudo seu whitmania*	*Shui zhi*
Lesser galangal rhizome	*Alpiniae officinari rizoma*	*Gao liang jiang*
Licorice root	*Glycyrrhizae uralensis radix*	*Gan cao*
Ligusticum root, Chinese lovage root	*Ligustici rhizoma et radix*	*Gao ben*
Ligustrum fruit	*Ligustri lucidi fructus*	*Nu zhen zi*
Lily bulb	*Lilii bulbus*	*Bai he*
Lindera root	*Linderae strychnifoliae radix*	*Wu yao*
Lithospermum, Groomwell root	*Arnebiae seu lithospermi radix*	*Zi cao*
Longan fruit	*Longanae arillus euphoriae*	*Long yan rou*
Loquat leaf	*Eriobotryae japonicae folium*	*Pi pa ye*
Loranthus branches	*Sangjisheng ramulus*	*Sang ji sheng*
Loranthus stem	*Loranthi ramulus*	*Sang ji sheng*
Lotus leaf	*Nelumbinis nuciferae folium*	*He ye*
Lotus seed	*Nelumbinis nuciferae semen*	*Lian zi*
Lotus stemen	*Nelumbinis nuciferae stamen*	*Lian xu*
Lycium berry, Wolfberry fruit	*Lycii chinensis fructus*	*Gou qi zi*
Lygodium spores	*Lygodii japonici herba*	*Hai jin sha*
Magnolia bark	*Magnoliae officinalis cortex*	*Hou po*
Magnolia flower	*Magnoliae liliflorae flos*	*Xin yi hua*
Magnolia flower	*Magnoliae flos*	*Hou po hua*
Maltose	*Saccharum granorum*	*Jiao yi*
Medicated leaven	*Massa fermenta*	*Shen qu*
Melia fruit	*Meliae toosendan fructus*	*Chuan lian zi*
Melon pedicle	*Cucumeris pedicellus*	*Gua di*
Mentha	*Mentha herba*	*Bo he*
Millettia root and vine, Chicken blood vine	*Jixueteng radix et caulis*	*Ji xue teng*

Common Name	Pharmaceutical	*Pin Yin*
Mimosa tree flower, Silk tree flower	*Albizziae julibrissin flos*	*He huan hua*
Mint	*Menthae haplocalycis herba*	*Bo he*
Mirabilite, Glauber's salt	*Mirabilitum*	*Mang xiao*
Mirabilite, Sodium sulphate	*Mirabilitum purum*	*Xuan ming fen*
Momordica Fruit	*Fructus Momordicae Grosvenori*	*Luo Han Guo*
Morinda root	*Morindae officinalis radix*	*Ba ji tian*
Morus bark, mulberry rootbark	*Mori albae radicis cortex*	*Sang bai pi*
Motherwort	*Leonuri heterophylli herba*	*Yi mu cao*
Mugwort leaf	*Artemisiae argyi folium*	*Ai ye*
Mulberry fruit bud	*Mori albae fructus*	*Sang shen*
Mulberry leaf	*Mori albae florium*	*Sang ye*
Mulberry mistletoe stems, loranthus	*Sangjisheng ramulus*	*Sang ji sheng*
Mulberry twig	*Mori albae ramulus*	*Sang zhi*
Mume, Black plum fruit	*Pruni mume*	*Wu mei*
Mung bean	*Phaseoli radiati semen*	*Lu dou*
Musk	*Moschus secretion*	*She xiang*
Myrrh	*Myrrha*	*Mo yao*
Notopterygium rhizome and root	*Notopterygii rhizoma et radix*	*Qiang huo*
Nut-grass rhizome, Cyperus	*Cyperi rotundi rhizoma*	*Xiang fu*
Oldenlandia	*Oldenlandiae diffusae herba*	*Bai hua she she cao*
Ophiopogon tuber, Creeping lily-turf tuber	*Ophiopogonis japonici tuber*	*Mai men dong*
Orthosiphon herb	*Orthosiphon herba*	*Hua shi cao*
Ox knee	*Achyranthis bidentatae radix*	*Niu xi*
Oyster shell	*Ostreae concha*	*Mu li*
Oyster shell calcined	*Concha ostreae*	*Duan mu li*
Pagoda tree flower bud	*Sophorae japonicae immaturus flos*	*Huai hua mi*
Pagoda tree fruit	*Sophorae japonicae fructus*	*Huai jiao*
Panax ginseng root (steamed until red)	*Ginseng radix*	*Ren shen hong*
Panax ginseng, Jilin wild ginseng	*Ginseng radix*	*Ji lin shen*

Common Name	Pharmaceutical	Pin Yin
Paris rhizome	Paridis rhizoma	Zao xiu
Patchouli, Agastache	Agastaches seu pogostemi herba	Huo xiang
Peach kernel	Persicae semen	Tao ren
Pearl	Margarita	Zhen zhu
Peony	Paeoniae radix	Shao yao
Perilla leaf	Perillae frutescentis folium	Zi su ye
Perilla leaf	Perillae frutescentis folium	Zi su ye
Perilla seed	Perillae frutescentis semen	Zi su zi
Perilla seed	Perillae frutescentis fructus	Su zi
Pinellia	Pinellia tuber	Ban xia
Pinellia rhizome	Pinelliae ternatae rhizoma	Ban xia (fa)
Plantago seed	Plantaginis semen	Che qian zi
Polygala Root	Radix Polygalae Tenuifoliae	Yuan Zhi
Polygonum	Polygoni perfoliati herba	Guan ye liao
Polyporus	Polypori umbellate sclerotium	Zhu ling
Praying mantis egg case	Mantidis ootheca	Sang piao xiao
Prepared Pinellia rhizome	Pinelliae tematae rhizome	Ban xia (sheng)
Prepared sichuan aconite root	Lateralis aconiti carmichaeli radix praeparata	Fu zi (hei)
Pseudoginseng root, notoginseng root	Pseudoginseng radix	San qi, (Tian qi)
Pueraria flower	Puerariae flos	Ge hua
Pulsatilla root	Pulsatillae chinensis radix	Bai tou weng
Pumice	Pumice	Fu hai shi
Purple aster root	Asteris tatarici radix	Zi wan
Pyrite	Pyritum	Zi ran tong
Pyrrosia leaf	Pyrrosiae folium	Shi wei
Rabdosia	Rabdosia rucescens	Dong ling cao
Radish seed	Raphani sativi semen	Lai fu zi
Realgar, Arsenic disulfide	Realgar	Xiong huang
Red date, Jujube fruit	Ziziphi jujubae fructus	Da zao
Red peony root	Paeoniae rubra radix	Chi shao
Red tangerine peel	Citri erythrocarpae pericarpium	Ju hong
Reed rhizome	Phragmitis communis rhizoma	Lu gen
Rhinoceros horn	Rhinoceri cornu	Xi jiao
Rhodioia herb	Rhodiola herba	Hong jing tian

Common Name	Pharmaceutical	Pin Yin
Rhododendron leaf	Rhodod foliumendri	Man shan hong
Rhubarb	Rhei rhizoma	Da huang
Rhubarb root	Rhei radix et rhizoma	Da huang
Rhubarb root	Rhei radix et rhizoma	Da huang
Rice grain	Oryzae sativae semen	Jing mi
Rice sprout	Oryzae sativae germinantus fructus	Gu ya
Rush pith	Junci effuse medulla	Deng xin cao
Safflower flower	Carthami tinctorii flos	Hong hua
Salvia	Salviae plebeya herba	Ji ning
Salvia root	Salviae miltiorrhizae radix	Dan shen
Sappan heartwood	Sappan lignum	Su mu
Saussurea	Natrium sulphuricum	Mu xiang
Schisandra fruit	Schisandrae chinensis fructus	Wu wei zi
Schizonepeta stem or bud	Schizonepetae tenuifoliae herba seu flos	Jing jie
Scophularia root, Figwort root	Scrophulariae ningpoensis radix	Xuan shen
Scuffy Pea	Psoraleae corylifoliae fructus	Bu gu zhi
Selfheal spike, Heal all spike	Prunellae vulgaris spica	Xia ku cao
Senna leaf	Sennae folium	Fan xie ye
Sesame	Sesami radix	Hu ma ren
Siberian Solomon seal rhizome	Polygonati rhizome	Huang jing
Sichuan ox knee root	Cyathulae radix	Chuan niu xi
Sichuan pepper seed	Zanthoxyli bungeani semen	Jiao mu (chuan)
Siler root	Ledebouriellae divaricatae radix	Fang feng
Siliceous secretions of bamboo	Bambusae textillis concretio silicea	Tian zhu huang
Silkworm feces	Bombycis mori excrementum	Can sha
Skullcap root, Scute	Scutellariae baicalensis radix	Huang qin
Smilax rhizome	Smilacis china rizoma	Ba qia
Smilax rhizome	Smilacis glabrae rhizoma	Tu fu ling
Snakegourd fruit	Trichosanthis fructus	Gua lou
Snakegourd peel	Trichosanthis pericarpium	Gua lou pi
Snakegourd root	Trichosanthis kirilowii radix	Tian hua fen
Snakegourd seed	Trichosanthis semen	Gua lou ren

Common Name	Pharmaceutical	Pin Yin
Solomon's Seal Rhizome, Polygonatum	*Polygonati odorati rhizoma*	*Yu zhu*
Sophora Root, Bitter ginseng root	*Sophorae flavescentis radix*	*Ku shen*
Sophora, Pigeon pea root	*Sophorae tokinensis radix*	*Shan dou gen*
Soybean prepared	*Sojae praeparatum semen*	*Dan dou chi*
Speranskia herb	*Speranskia tuberculata*	*Tou gu cao*
St. john's wort	*Hypericum perforatum*	*Tian ji huang*
Star jasmine stem	*Tracachelospermi jasminoidis caulis*	*Luo shi teng*
Stephania root	*Stephaniae tetrandrae radix*	*Han fang ji*
Styrax benzoin processed resin	*Benzoinum*	*An xi xiang*
Sulphur	*Sulphur*	*Liu huang*
Szechuan lovage root	*Ligustici chuanxiong radix*	*Chuan xiong*
Talc, Soapstone	*Talcum*	*Hua shi*
Tang kuei head	*Angelicae sinensis caput radicis*	*Dang gui tou*
Tang kuei root	*Angelicae sinensis radix*	*Dang gui*
Tang kuei tail	*Angelicae sinensis extremas radicis*	*Dang gui wei*
Tangerine peel	*Citri reticulatae pericarpium*	*Chen pi*
Tangerine seed	*Citri reticulatae semen*	*Ju he*
Tea	*Camelliae folium*	*Cha ye*
Thiaspi, Patrinia	*Patriniae heterophyllae herba*	*Bai jiang cao*
Thin cinnamon bark form young trees	*Cinnamomi cassiae cortex tubiformis*	*Guan gui*
Tokoro, Yam rhizome	*Dioscorae hypoglaucae rhizome*	*Bei xie*
Tree peony root-bark	*Moutan radicis cortex*	*Mu dan pi*
Tricosanthes root	*Trichosanthis radix*	*Gua lou gen*
Tuckahoe skin	*Poriae cocos cortex*	*Fu ling pi*
Tuckahoe spirit	*Poriae cocos sclerotium pararadicis*	*Fu shen*
Tumeric tuber	*Curcumae tuber*	*Yu jin*
Turmeric rhizome	*Curcumae rhizoma*	*Jiang huang*
Vervain leaf	*Verbenae herba*	*Ma bian cao*
Vitex fruit	*Viticis fructus*	*Man jing zi*
Vladimiria root	*Vladimiriae radix*	*Chuan mu xiang*

Common Name	Pharmaceutical	*Pin Yin*
Water plantain rhizome	*Alismatis orientalis rhizoma*	*Ze xie*
White Atractylodes root	*Atractylodis macrocephalae rhizoma*	*Bai zhu*
White Peony root	*Paeoniae lactiflorae radix*	*Bai shao*
Wild Chrysanthemum flower	*Chrysanthemi indici flos*	*Ye ju hua*
Wild ginseng	*Ginseng radix*	*Ye shan shen*
Wild yam	*Dioscoreae oppositae radix*	*Shan yao*
Wine cooked rehmannia, Foxglove	*Rehmanniae glutinosae conquitae radix*	*Shu di huang*
Woad root	*Isatidis seu baphicacanthi radix*	*Ban lan gen*
Wolfberry root cortex	*Lycii chinensis radicis cortex*	*Di gu pi*
Xanthium, Cocklebur fruit	*Xanthii fructus*	*Cang er zi*
Yedeon's Violet	*Violae cum radice herba*	*Zi hua di ding*
Zanthoxylum, Sichuan pepper fruit	*Zanthoxyli pericarpium bungeani*	*Chuan jiao*
Zedoary rhizome, Tumeric rhizome	*Curcumae rhizoma*	*E zhu*
Zizyphus seed, Sour jujube	*Zizyphi spinosae semen*	*Suan zao ren*

Classification and Function (Herb List)

Pin Yin	Pharmaceutical	Herb Classification	Herb Function
Ba dou	Crotonis semen	Purgatives	Purge cold stagnation
Bai zhi	Angelicae dahurica radix	Exterior-releasing (pungent-warm)	Disperse wind and pain (such as stuffy nose and headache), eliminate damp-heat (i.e. leukorrhalgia), discharges pus and reduces, swelling at the surface
Bai zhu	Atractylodis macrocephalae rhizoma	Tonics	Replenish qi, tonify the spleen arrest excessive sweating, and calm the fetus
Bai zi ren	Biotae orientalis semen	Sedatives	Nourishes heart Yin and heart blood
Ban xia (fa)	Pinelliae ternatae rhizoma	Antittussives, Expectorants, and antithmatics (resolve cold-phlegm)	Expectorant (cough with thin-white phlegm), antiemetic
Bei mu	Fritillariae bulbus	Antitussives	Clears heat and resolves thick phlegm, reduces nodules in mastitis and scrofula
Bing lang	Arecae catechu semen	Anthelmintic	Removes undigested food and ascarasis, induces diuresis, and arrests malarial episodes
Bo he	Menthae herba	Exterior-releasing (pungent cool)	Disperses wind-heat, Clears the head and eyes, promotes eruptions of measles, Soothes the liver
Cang zhu	Atractylodis rizoma	Fragrant herbs that resolve dampness	Supplement the stomach and spleen, resolve dampness, dispel wind-damp

Pin Yin	Pharmaceutical	Herb Classification	Herb Function
Cha ye	Camelliae folium	Diuretics	Resolves phlegm, removes toxins and stagnant food, promotes diuresis
Chai hu	Bupleuri radix	Exterior-releasing (pungent-cool)	Reduce fever (alternating chills and fever), relieve liver qi stagnation, lift spleen qi
Chan tui	Cicadae periostracum	Exterior-releasing (pugent-cooling)	Disperses wind-heat, promotes eruptions of measles and relieves itching, improves eye sight, relieves spasms in infantile convulsion
Che qian zi	Plantaginis semen	Diuretics	Increases urination, clears the liver and improves vision, resolves lung phlegm
Chen pi	Citri reticulatae pericarpium	Regulates qi flow	Regulates qi, supplements spleen, dispels dampness and resolves phlegm
Chi shao	Paeoniae rubra radix	Blood regulating	Invigorates and cools blood
Chi shi zhi	Halloysitum rubrum	Astringents and Hemostatics	Astringe bloody stool
Chi xiao dou	Phaseoli calcarati semen	Diuretics	Promotes diuresis, reduces heat and swelling, moves blood
Chuan jiao	Zanthoxyli pericarpium bungeani	Interior warming	Warms and dispels dampness in the spleen and stomach, controls abdominal pain, and kills ascarids
Chuan xiong	Ligustici chuanxiong radix	Activate blood and resolve stasis	Promotes the flow of qi and blood, Dispels wind and relieves pain
Da huang	Rhei radix et rhizoma	Purgatives	Clears heat, purges toxic heat, and removes blood stasis

Pin Yin	Pharmaceutical	Herb Classification	Herb Function
Da zao	Ziziphi jujubae fructus	Tonics	Supplements qi and blood
Dan dou chi	Sojae praeparatum semen	Exterior-releasing (pungent-cool)	Used in the early stage of febrile disease to relieve the surface and late stage to relieve fidgetiness and insomnia
Dan shen	Salviae miltiorrhizae radix	Activate blood and resolve stasis	Move blood and resolve blood stasis, clear heat in the blood, and calm the heart
Dang gui	Angelicae sinensis radix	Blood tonics	Nourishes and activates the blood, emollient and laxative
Dong gua zi	Benincasae semen	Diuretics	Induce diuresis
Du huo	Angelicae pubescentis radix	Dispels wind-damp	Dispels wind-cold and wind-damp, mainly in the lower jiao
E jiao	Asini cori gelatinum	Blood tonics	Nourishes the blood, arrest bleeding, and tonifies the yin
Fang feng	Ledebouriellae divaricatae radix	Exterior-releasing (pungent-warm)	Dispels wind-damp in cases of urticaria, dispels wind-damp and pain in cases of rheumatalgia
Fu ling	Poriae cocos sclerotium	Diuretics	Diuretic, supplements spleen function, helps tranquilize heart palpitations
Fu zi (hei)	Lateralis aconiti carmichaeli radix praeparata	Dispels internal cold	Dispels cold and restores heart, kidney, and spleen yang
Gan cao	Glycyrrhizae uralensis radix	Tonics	Replenish qi, tonify the spleen and heart, clear the meridians to reduce pain, and counteract toxins
Gan jiang	Zingiberis officinalis rhizoma	Dispels internal cold	Warms the spleen, stomach, and lungs

Pin Yin	Pharmaceutical	Herb Classification	Herb Function
Gan sui	Euphorbiae kansui radix	Purgatives	Dispels fluid, purges water toxins, and reduces swelling
Ge gen	Puerariae radix	Exterior-releasing (pungent-cool)	Reduce fever, eliminates pain in the neck and upper back, relieves thirst, promotes eruption of measles, arrest diarrhea
Gou teng	Uncariae cum uncis ramulus	Spasmolytics	Calms the liver-wind, clears heat, controls convulsions
Gua di	Cucumeris pedicellus	Emetics	Induces expectoration and vomiting of undigested food
Gua lou gen	Trichosanthis radix	Antititussives, Expectorants, and antithmatics (resolve hot-phlegm)	Clears heat and resolves phlegm, soothes chest pain related to angina pectoris, moistens the bowels, and treats lung abscess
Gua lou ren	Trichosanthis semen	Cool and transform hot phlegm	Clears hot phlegm, promotes qi circulation in upper jiao and the healing of sores
Gui zhi	Cinnamomi cassiae ramulus	Exterior-releasing (pungent-warm)	Control sweating caused by wind-cold invasion, warm and unblock the meridians, Stimulate menstruation
Hou po	Magnoliae officinalis cortex	Aromatic and drying	Dries dampness in spleen and stomach, reduces inflammation, and moves qi stagnation
Hu huang lian	Picrohizae	Clear heat and dry dampness	Clears damp-heat resulting in acute dysentery and jaundice
Hu ma ren	Sesami radix	Purgatives	Moistens dryness, helps clear the intestines, and nourishes liver-blood and kidneys

Pin Yin	*Pharmaceutical*	Herb Classification	Herb Function
Hua shi	Talcum	Diuretics	Clears summer-heat and dispels dampness in the lower *jiao*
Huang bai	Phellodendri cortex	Clear heat and dry dampness	Clears damp-heat, high fever that causes dysentery jaundice, mobid leukorrhea, and yin deficiency
Huang lian	Coptidis rhizoma	Clear heat and dry dampness	Clears damp-heat, high fever that causes dysentery and skin boils
Huang qi	Astragali membranaceus radix	Tonics	Tonifies spleen qi, expels pus and accelerates healing of chronic ulcers
Huang qin	Scutellariae baicalensis radix	Clear heat and dry dampness	Clears damp-heat, clears toxic heat that cause boils and skin sores, cools blood and helps prevent miscarriage
Jiao yi	Saccharum granorum	Tonics	Supplements spleen and stomach, moistens the lungs, and controls pain
Jie geng (ku)	Platycodi grandiflori radix	Antitussives	Resolves cold-phlegm in the upper *jiao*, soothes the throat, and drains pus
Jin yin hua	Lonicerae japonicae flos	Clear heat toxins	Clears wind-heat and toxic-heat
Jing jie	Schizonepetae tenuifoliae herba seu flos	Exterior-releasing (pungent-warm)	Disperses wind-cold, promotes eruptions (measles)
Jing mi	Oryzae sativae semen	Digestive	Improves digestion
Ku shen	Sophorae flavescentis radix	Clear heat and dry dampness	Clears damp-heat and kills parasitic worms
Lei wan	Omphaliae scierotium lapidescens	Anthelmintic	Kills intestinal parasites
Lian jiao	Forsythiae fructus	Febrifuges	Dispels toxic heat, reduces swellings, and drains pus

Pin Yin	Pharmaceutical	Herb Classification	Herb Function
Long dan cao	Gentianae longdancao radix	Clear heat and dry dampness	Clears damp-heat in liver and gallbladder, liver fire with hyperchondriac pain and headache
Long gu	Os draconis	Sedatives	Subdues excess yang, pacifies liver yang
Ma huang	Epherdrae herba	Exterior-releasing (pungent-warm)	Induce sweating for wind-cold conditions, relieve asthma, induce diuresis for relieveing edema caused by wind envasion
Mai men dong	Ophiopogonis japonici tuber	Yin tonics	Replenishes and promotes fluid production, nourishes the stomach yin and lung yin, and calms the mind
Mang xiao	Mirabilitum	Purgatives	Purges toxins and externally softens hard masses related to acute mastitis
Meng chong	Tabani Bivittati	Activate blood and resolve stasis	Remove severe blood stasis, dissolve swelling
Mu dan pi	Moutan radicis cortex	Clear Heat and Cool Blood	Febrile diseases with eruptions and bleeding, activate blood circulation and removes stasis
Mu li	Ostreae concha	Sedatives	Softens and disperses hard lumps, nourishes the yin
Mu tong	Mutong caulis	Diuretics	Resolves damp-heat in the lower *jiao*
Mu xiang	Natrium sulphuricum	Qi regulating	Promotes qi circulation, controls pain and diarrhea, and relieves abdominal distention

Pin Yin	Pharmaceutical	Herb Classification	Herb Function
Niu bang zi	Arctii lappae fructus	Exterior-releasing (pugent-cooling)	Disperses wind-heat, promotes eruptions of measles, counteracts toxins and reduces swelling at the surface
Qian hu	Peucedani radix	Antitussives	Resolves phlegm-heat and helps qi to descend, disperses wind-heat
Qiang huo	Notopterygii rhizoma et radix	Dispels wind-damp	Dispels wind-cold and wind-damp mainly in the upper part of the body
Ren shen	Ginseng radix	Tonics	Supplements qi and promotes fluid production, tonifies lungs and spleen, and nourishes heart yin
Sang bai pi	Mori albae radicis cortex	Antitussives	Purge lung heat, induce diarrhea in case of edema
Shan jiao	Zanthoxyli pericarpium bungeani	Interior warming	Warms and dispels dampness in the spleen and stomach, controls abdominal pain, and kills ascarids
Shao yao	Paeoniae radix	Blood regulating	Invigorates and cools blood
Sheng di huang	Rehmanniae glutinosae radix	Febrifuges	Cools blood, controls bleeding, nourishes yin and blood
Sheng jiang	Zingiberis officinalis recens rhizoma	Exterior-releasing (pungent-warm)	Induce sweating for wind-cold conditions, warm the middle *jiao* and arrest vomiting
Sheng ma	Cimicifugae rhizoma	Exterior-releasing (pungent-cooling)	Promotes eruption of measles, clears heat and counteracts toxins in the upper *jiao*, help restore the normal position of prolapsed organs

Pin Yin	*Pharmaceutical*	Herb Classification	Herb Function
Shi chang pu	Acori graminei rhizoma	Aromatic stimulant	Resolves dampness and harmonizes the stomach, treats impaired consciousness
Shi gao	Gypsum fibrosum	Clear Heat, Fire Purging	Dispels high fever, dispels heat in lungs and stomach, and externally, promotes the healing of wounds and ulcers
Shou di huang	Rehmanniae glutinosae conquitae radix	Tonic	Tonifies the blood and kidney yin
Shui zhi	Hirudo seu whitmania	Activate blood and resolve stasis	Remove severe blood stasis, dissolve swelling
Suan zao ren	Zizyphi spinosae semen	Sedatives	Supplements the yin and arrests excessive sweating
Suo sha	Amoni semen	Aromatic and drying	Moves and regulates qi flow, clears food stagnation in the stomach, prevents spontaneous abortion
Tao ren	Persicae semen	Activate blood and resolve stasis	Promote blood flow and remove stasis
Tian men dong	Asparagi cochinchinensis tuber	Tonics	Nourishes yin, clears lung fire, and controls dry cough
Wu mei	Pruni mume	Astringents and Hemostatics	Antidiarrhetic, antitussive, antidiptic, and antithelmetic
Wu wei zi	Schisandrae chinensis fructus	Astringents and Hemostatics	Astringent and a tranquilizer for palpitations and insomnia
Wu zhu yu	Evodiae rutaecarpae fructus	Dispels internal cold	Warms the stomach
Xi xin	Asari herba radice	Exterior-releasing (pungent-warm)	Dispels wind and cold, warms the lungs and resolves retained fluid

Pin Yin	Pharmaceutical	Herb Classification	Herb Function
Xiang fu zi	Cyperi rotundi rhizoma	Qi regulating	Regulates liver qi stagnation, regulates menses, and controls pain
Xie bai	Allii bulbus macrostemi	Qi regulating	Dispels cold and regulates qi stagnation in the upper jiao, promotes yang, and moistens the intestines
Xing ren	Pruni armeniacae semen	Antitussives	Controls cough, moistens lungs and intestines, and promotes bowel movement
Xuan shen	Scrophulariae ningpoensis radix	Clear Heat and Cool Blood	Clears heat, cools the blood, and replenishes yin; for treatment at the ying (nutritive) level of disease
Yan hu suo	Corydalis rhizome Yanhusuo	Blood regulating	Controls pain, invigorates blood, increases qi circulation
Yi yi ren	Coicis lachryma-jobi	Diuretics	Invigorates the spleen and clears damp-heat, discharge pus form lungs
Yin chen hao	Artemisiae yinchenhao herba	Clear heat and dry dampness	Clears damp-heat in liver and gallbladder, liver fire with hyperchondriac pain and jaundice
Yuan Zhi	Radix Polygalae Tenuifoliae	Sedatives	Expels phlegm, reduces toxic heat, nourishes the yin
Ze xie	Alismatis orientalis rhizoma	Diyretic	Clears damp-heat in lower jiao
Zhi ke	Citri aurantii fructus	Qi regulating	Dissolves phlegm, disperses qi stagnation, and dissipates fullness in all three jiaos

Pin Yin	Pharmaceutical	Herb Classification	Herb Function
Zhi mu	Anemarrhenae asphodeloidis radix	Febrifuges	Relieves thirst and high fever, nourishes the yin and kidneys
Zhi shi	Citri seu ponciri immaturus fructus	Qi regulating	Moves and regulates qi flow, clears food stagnation in the stomach
Zhi zi	Gardenia jasminoidis fructus	Clear heat and dry dampness	Purges fire and calms the mind, Clears damp-heat in liver and gallbladder, and cools blood toxins
Zhu li	Bambusae succus	Cool and transform hot phlegm	Clears heat and resolves hot-phlegm, alleviates cough
Zhu ling	Polypori umbellati sclerotium	Diuretics	Diuretic and clears damp heat in the lower jiao
Zhu ru	Bambusae in taenilis caulis	Antititussives, Expectorants, and antithmatics (resolve hot-phlegm)	Clears damp-heat and vomiting due to stomach heat
Zhu sha	Cinnabaris	Sedatives	Treats palpitations, insomnia, infantile convulsion, epilepsy, and clears toxic heat
Zhu ye	Bambusae folium	Febrifuges	Clears damp-heat, releases exterior wind-heat, promotes urination, lessens irritability
Zi su ye	Perillae frutescentis semen	Exterior-releasing (pungent-warm)	Induces sweating to treat wind-cold, arrest vomiting, an antidote for fish and crab poisoning

Bibliography

Chinese Herbal Medicine Materia Medica. (1986). (D. Bensky, A. Gamble, & T. Kaptchuk, Trans.) Seattle, Wa: Eastland Press.

Bingshan, H. (n.d.). *Syndromes of Tradtional Chinese Medicine Analysis of 338 Syndromes.* (W. Donou'en, S. Shuangli, & C. Honxin, Trans.) Jiuzhan, Daoli, Harbin, China: Heilongjiang Education Press.

The Nei Ching (Su Wen, and Ling Shu, and Nan Ching) Chinese Medical Classics. (1979, December). *Limited Edition.* (A. Chamfrault, N. Van Nghi, Trans., & M. Barnett, Compiler) Miami, Florida, USA: Occidental Institute of Chinese Studies Alumni Association.

Hsu, H.-y. (1983). *Chin Kuei Yao Lueh.* (H.-Y. Hsu, & S.-Y. Wang, Trans.) Long Beach, Ca: Oriental Healing Arts Institute.

Hsu, H.-y. (1984). An Outline of Oriental Materia Medica. *Bulletin of the Oriental Healing Arts Institute of U.S.A.*

Hsu, H.-y., & Hsu, C.-s. (1980). *Commonly Used Chinese Herb Formulas.* Long beach, Ca: Oriental Healing Arts Institute.

Hsu, H.-y., & Hsu, C.-s. (1990). *Commonly Used Chinese Herb Formulas With Illustrations Companion Handbook.* Long Beach, Ca: Oriental Healing Arts Institute.

Hsu, H.-y., & Peacher, W. (1981). *Shang Han Lun The Great Classic of Chinese Medicine.* Long Beach, Ca: OHAI.

Hsu, H.-y., Chen, Y.-p., Sheu, S.-j., Hsu, C.-s., Chen, C.-c., & Chang, H.-c. (1986). *Oreintal Materia Medica: A Concise Guide.* Lon Beach, Ca: Oriental Healing Arts Institute.

Moore, J. M. (1995). *Shang Han Lun and Other Traditional Formulas.* Long Beach, Ca: Oriental Healing Arts Institute.

Otsuka, K., Yakazu, D., Shimizu, T., & Hsu, H.-y. (1982). *Natural Healing With Chinese Herbs*. (Hsu-Hong-yen, Ed.) Los Angeles, Ca: Oiental Healing Arts Intitute.

Xie, Z.-F. (2002). *Classified Dictionary of Traditional Chineser Medicne* (New Edition ed.). Beijing, China: Forein Languages Press, Beijing.